Spoken English

"A Practical Course for Speaking English Correctly & Effectively"

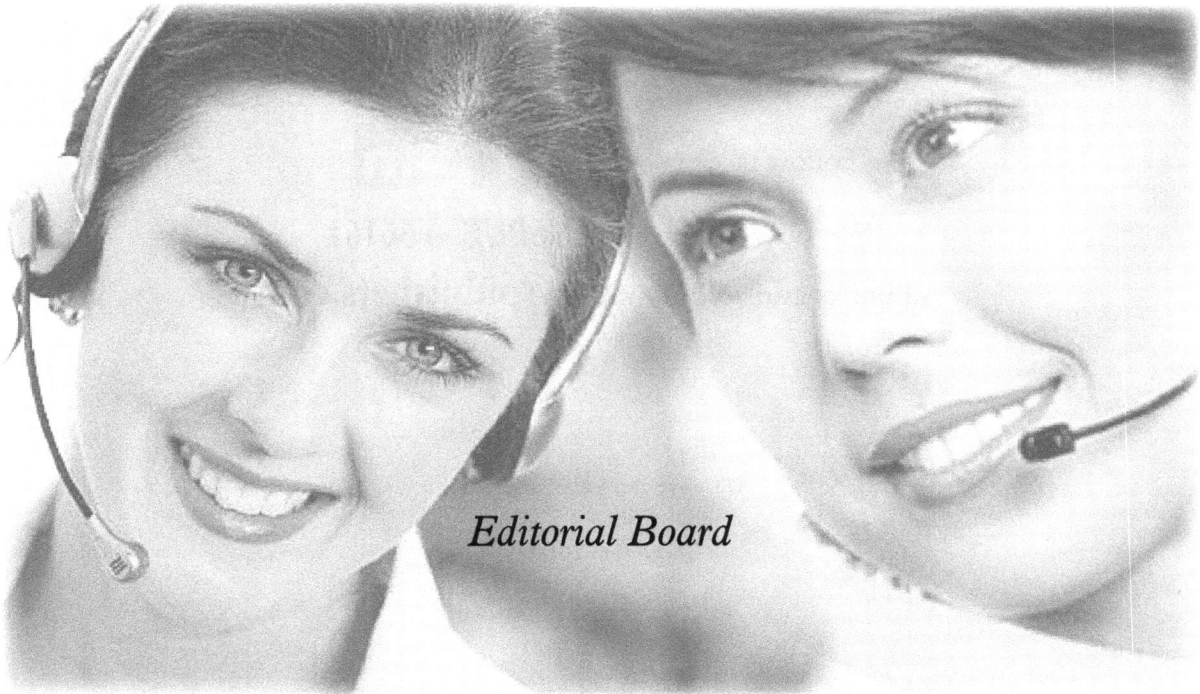

Editorial Board

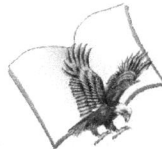

V&S PUBLISHERS

Published by:

V&S PUBLISHERS

F-2/16, Ansari Road, Daryaganj, New Delhi-110002
☎ 011-23240026, 011-23240027 • *Fax:* 011-23240028
Email: info@vspublishers.com • *Website:* www.vspublishers.com

Branch : Hyderabad
5-1-707/1, Brij Bhawan (Beside Central Bank of India Lane)
Bank Street, Koti, Hyderabad - 500 095
☎ 040-24737290
E-mail: vspublishershyd@gmail.com

Follow us on: 🐦 f in

For any assistance sms **VSPUB** to **56161**

All books available at **www.vspublishers.com**

Printed at : Unique Colour Carton, New Delhi-110020

PUBLISHER'S NOTE

It has been our prime motto and a constant endeavour at **V&S Publishers** to publish books of **Value** and **Substance** from the time of its inception. With a backlist of **about 350 titles** to our credit, it's a great pleasure to inform all our esteemed readers that we have come up with this altogether exclusive series of books on **English language and its various usage** called the **EXC-EL Series – Excellence in English Language Series**.

The series contains a set of books on *various usage of* Words and Phrases in English, the significance of Grammar, correct Pronunciation, etc., called *English Grammar And Usage, English Vocabulary made Easy, Improve Your Vocabulary* and *Spoken English* to enhance and enrich your vocabulary, increase your command over the language and make you more confident and fluent in your day to day conversations, written and verbal interactions, etc.

The present book, ***Spoken English*** broadly deals with the four basic aspects of English language – *Grammar, Pronunciation, Conversation* and *Vocabulary*. Understanding and learning each of these aspects is equally important for speaking and writing correct and good English. All these aspects have been elaborately discussed in the book with ample Examples and Exercises to help layman and the students to get a grasp of the language and master it. The fact that no second language has been used gives it a universal appeal.

While the Grammar section focuses on selective aspects which are important form Spoken English point of view and in short explains the concept, the pronunciation section is unique in its own way and without technical jargon helping readers to speak English correctly and fluently.

The section on conversation has numerous conversations from day to day life to help readers get a feel of Spoken English. All conversations are simple and to the point for ease in understanding.

An additional section on vocabulary is appended at the end which makes this book a one-stop solution for anyone and everyone who intends to learn English, especially Spoken English.

We hope the book will be beneficial to readers of all ages, particularly the student section and will serve its purpose well.

CONTENTS

SECTION 4 : VOCABULARY

AN INTRODUCTION

With the globalisation of knowledge and culture the need for acquiring good communicative English by one and all has assumed great significance in this twenty first century. In fact, the demand for learning effective communicative English has never been as great as it stands today. It is interesting to note that during the last two decades the use of English for communicative purposes has not been confined only to the elite group of the society. People from the middle and lower middle classes are equally keen on learning and using it effectively.

It is because they consider 'Spoken English' as a passport for a guaranteed success in life. The craze for learning Spoken English has led to the growth of various coaching institutes all over the country. Much as they may profess and advertise it is not really possible to learn any language in thirty or forty days. At the same time learning Spoken English does not mean parrot like repetition of some crammed sentences with the help of a limited vocabulary. It means acquiring a skill to generate and use functional English in ever changing life situations while speaking. For this besides acquiring the required sentence patterns and expressions in a given situation a person needs an appropriate vocabulary as well. So this is surely not possible in two or three month's time. Although one needs to understand that a person who genuinely wants to learn the language needs to spend at least two to three hours every day for at least five or six months before he or she feels confident to communicate in English. A strong desire coupled with one track working is a pre condition for the successful completion of this project on communicative English.

In India, as everywhere, English offers its own problems. It becomes a language of 'iffs and butts' where double 'f's and double't's crop up at the most unlikely of places giving emphasis where there should be subtlety. Caught between the inability to articulate in a foreign language and the rather inexplicable need to be seen using English, the Indian actually gets the shivers. Over the years with mobile phones and computers spreading all over India, the country's fascination with English ahs only intensified. It cannot be said for sure if this has resulted in English usage getting more communicative. At the moment the process is a bit haphazard and finding a method in this madness is the idea of this book.

The objective of this book is to encourage students & layman to learn English as a tool of communication and to enable them 'to know, to do, to live and to live.' It looks at language from the learner's point of view and guides them through co-operative learning methods in order to master effective communication skills.

The goal of teaching speaking skills is communicative efficiency. Learners should be able to make themselves understood, using their current proficiency to the fullest. They should try to avoid confusion in the message due to faulty pronunciation, grammar, or vocabulary, and to observe the social and cultural rules that apply in each communication situation.

The book is divided into convenient units. Each chapter covers one main area of learning English with special attention given to basic skills. Carefully selected, balanced practical exercises are designed to give practice in form, meaning and use of English. The book follows modern functional approach to the study of English.

Although there are a few books available in the market on Spoken English they do not really help an individual acquire the communicative skills. They primarily deal with technical knowledge and the accompanying jargons. The section of grammar and usage I each chapter of this book provides necessary help to a learner for the understanding of certain grammatical points appearing in spoken English. Besides dealing with situations from day to day life the book also attempts to provide its users with the essentials of spoken English required to speak English with confidence.

Knowing the Two Mediums: Speech and Writing

Speech and writing are the two mediums of language. The sounds of speech and the letters of writing are in themselves meaningless, but they are combined according to the underlying system of language to convey specific meanings and perform specific functions. As mediums, speech and writing are concrete, whereas the underlying system of language is abstract.

In terms of physical features, speech consists of sounds that are perceived by the ear and is therefore ephemeral, whereas writing consists of marks on a surface that are perceived by the eye and is therefore permanent.

Though speech and writing function independently as medium of language, it is possible to transfer speech into writing and vice versa, because writing is a symbolic representation of speech.

As there are striking discrepancies between pronunciation and spelling, particularly in a language like English, it is important to study each medium independently and not transfer the features of one to another.

The characteristic features of speech and writing make them suitable for different communicative functions. As writing can be preserved for long periods of time and can also be transported across long distances, it is used more frequently than speech to convey factual information. Similarly, because speech is more suited to face-to-face communication, it is used more frequently than writing for interpersonal functions. Further, as writing is more resistant to changes with time and also more homogeneous; it is preferred in all the prestigious activities of society like administration, education, trade, law, etc.

Each of the two mediums has its advantages. Writing, as the more stable medium preserves much historical, lexical, morphological and grammatical information that is lost in speech. Also, when writing a person can read over what she has written and correct and revise if necessary which is not possible when speaking. A reader can choose what to read, whereas in speech a listener does not have this kind of choice.

Speech is characterized by features like variations in pitch, stress and voice quality and is accompanied by facial expression and gestures, all of which convey meanings additional to those of the actual words used. Speech also has the advantage of immediate feedback from the listener/s, so that the speaker can make her speech both accessible and acceptable to the listeners.

Let us consider two examples, one of speech, and the other of writing that will make clear the differences between the two mediums in the way they use language. Both these examples describe a rainbow, but in different ways.

First the sample of spoken language:

You see+ well+ er+ a series of stripes+ formed like a bow+ an arch+ very very far away+ ah+ seven colours but+ I guess you hardly ever see seven it's just a + series of + colours which…

Which we find here are sequences of phrases and clauses and not complete and finished sentences. Spoken language is also characterized by repetition as in a series of stripes and series of colours, use of markers of hesitation like ah, er, etc and monitoring devices like you see.

Now, let's look at the sample of written language:

In one place it gleamed fiercely, and her heart anguished with hope, she sought the shadow of iris where the bow should be. Steadily the colour gathered mysteriously from nowhere, it took presence upon itself; there was a faint, vast rainbow. (G.Brown and G. Yule, discourse Analysis)

Here we have complete sentences that are clearly marked by capital letters and full stops. Also the structures used are quite complex.

Another important difference between speech and writing is that speech is prior to writing a medium of language. The priority of speech over writing can be explained in historical structural, functional and biological terms. Historically, writing is only a few thousand years old, whereas man has been known to speak language from much earlier ages. Also, human beings learn to speak before they learnt to read or write. Structurally, speech is more basic than writing because writing is a symbolic representation of speech. In terms of use too, speech has acquired priority over writing as it is used for a wider range of purposes than writing. With the advent of recording devices, speech has become as permanently preservable as only writing once was. Further, biologically, the left part of the brain that processes language, i.e. the left hemisphere, which is more dominant than the right one in most people, is better at processing speech sounds.

Organisation of the Book

Section one is **English Grammar** and this discusses the grammatical points arising out of a given model conversation. The learner is expected to go through them carefully to acquire correctness of speech, with fluency in his or her communication. As a thumb rule, it is good to remember that where there is a conflict between a grammatical rule and a usage; preference should be given to the usage. The preference for usage will help the learners use English as a living language.

Section two is **Pronunciation** and the following areas of:

a. English sounds,

b. Word stress

c. Sentence stress

d. Intonation

The important aspects of pronunciation has been touched upon which should enable the learner to assimilate and comprehend the need for clear pronunciation and cogent enunciation of words for better communication.

Section three is **Conversation** and this presents a model conversation in a given situation. The learner is expected to read it aloud alone, or with the help of his or her friend to know how he/she sounds while communicating in English. Ideally it should be read aloud by two or more persons depending on the number of characters involved in the conversation. But when it not feasible, for any reason, an individual may read aloud the dialogues of all the characters as well. Believe me the result will be equally profitable.

Section four is **Vocabulary**, as we all know that learning a language is incomplete without Vocabulary which is nothing but a set of words within a language that a person is familiar with.

However, with **age** and **good education**, usually the vocabulary of a person keeps on developing and becomes more and more extensive, polished and powerful. This, in turn strengthens, one's hold over a language increasing one's writing and speaking skills in that language.

In this section, there are *Antonyms, Synonyms, Homonyms, Homophones, Prefixes, Suffixes, Idioms, Proverbs, Phrases*, etc., all with lots of **Examples** and **Exercises** to make you easily understand and enrich your vocabulary enhancing your command over the English language.

Section 1
English Grammar

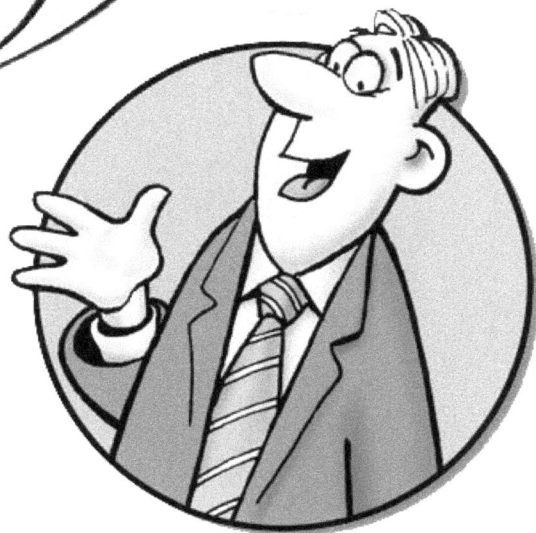

GRAMMATICAL FEATURES

Grammatical Features are features that characterize specific categories or classes of grammatical units like noun, verbs, noun phrases, verb phrases etc. these classes of words and phrases also differ in terms of specific grammatical features which characterize them. Nouns and noun phrases are described in terms of features like number (singular, girl, or plural, girls) and case (Nominative, girl, or genitive, girl's), whereas verbs and verb phrases are described in terms of features like tense (present, go, or past, went), aspect (perfective, has gone, or non-perfective, go). These grammatical features represent another type of grammatical choices that we make in combining words into longer units. In a clause like I have seen these new books in the library, for example, we saw that the second position that of the verb phrase have seen, can be filled by other verb phrases like saw will see, can borrow, like and have read. These examples show that there are two types of choice possible, one, the choice between verbs like see, borrow, like and read and the other, between verb phrases with the same verb see like saw and will see, which differ from have seen in tense and aspect or in modality. The first is a choice between different vocabulary items, whereas the second is a choice between different grammatical features. Thus, in any given position in a grammatical unit, two grammatical choices are made, choice of the constituent from the appropriate grammatical class and choice of appropriate grammatical feature/s characteristic of the class to which the chosen constituent belongs.

We know the choice of appropriate constituents, determines whether the combination of words is grammatical or not and also the meaning it conveys. The second type of choice, the choice of the appropriate grammatical feature/s with the constituents, is also equally important in deciding the grammaticality and the meaning of the combination of words. For example, in the noun phrase these new books, it is not only necessary to choose a noun in the position filled by books. It is equally important that we choose the plural form of the noun. Thus, if we choose other nouns like pen, journal, toy, car, etc, for this position, we have to choose the plural forms of these nouns pens, journals, toys, cars etc. The choice of the singular form will result in an ungrammatical combination as in

These new pen

These new journal

These new toy

These new car

We see that this is because the determiner in position 1, *these*, is plural and the number of the noun chosen in position 3 must agree with the number of the determiner in position 1. If we make a different choice in position 1 and have the in place of these, it is possible to have either the singular or the plural form of the noun in position 3, because the can be used either with singular or plural nouns. In this case, the choice between the singular or plural noun will result in difference of meaning as in

The new book	the new books
The new pen	the new pens
The new journal	the new journals
The new toy	the new toys
The new car	the new cars

There are different means by which choices of grammatical features are indicated. In order to mark the plural form of nouns we add a suffix-s or –es (pronounced /s/, /z/ or /Iz/) in most cases. In case of verbs we add the suffix-ed (pronounced /t/, /d/ or /Id/) to mark the past tense in most cases, as in

They type letters.

They typed letters.

But in order to indicate the perfective aspect, we make two changes, use the auxiliary verb have and also add the suffix-ex. Thus in

They play tennis

If we have to change the aspect of the verb play from non-perfective to perfective, play becomes have played and we will have

They have played tennis.

Similarly, if we wish to change the modality of the verb, we add a modal auxiliary before the verb as in

They may go home.

They can go home.

They must go home.

They will go home.

Auxiliary verbs like have and modal auxiliaries like may, can, will and must are used on ly to perform these important grammatical functions of marking the perfective aspect and the modality of verbs and always occur with full verbs like type, play etc. they do not have independent meanings and cannot be used by themselves. They are, therefore called grammatical words in contrast to full verbs like type and play which have independent meanings and which are called lexical words.

Thus, we have mainly two devices, the addition of a suffix and the use of a grammatical word like an auxiliary verb, by which we mark grammatical features like number and case with nouns, and tense, aspect and modality and verbs.

Grammar and Meaning

Grammar helps us to combine words in different ways to communicate different meanings. When we consider the relationship between grammar and meaning, we notice the grammar is used to convey different types of meaning.

1. Generally, when we think of meaning, we think of ideas, facts, thoughts, beliefs etc. This is one type of meaning, which can be called conceptual or factual meaning. It is obvious that grammar plays a very important role in conveying conceptual or factual meaning. The following are a

few examples of this role of grammar.

She ordered a book. The book was delivered to her the next day.

She ordered a book. A book was delivered to her the next day.

In the first sentence the use of the shows that the book that was delivered to her was the same book that she ordered. But in the second sentence, the use of the article a questions whether it was the same book or not. In fact, it may suggest that it was not the same book.

He found the old man's shoes.

He found the man's old shoes.

The difference in the sequence in which the two words old and man's occur results in the difference in meaning between the two sentences.

Young people love music and dancing.

Young people loved music and dancing

Young people may love music and dancing.

Here the difference in tense between the first and the second sentences marks a difference in time reference. In the third sentence it is the use of the modal auxiliary may which makes it suggest a sense of possibility.

Children love animals.

Animals love children.

The two words children and animals occur in different positions and have different grammatical functions in the two sentences, and therefore, the two sentences have different meanings.

The policeman in the blue car shot the bandit.

The policeman shot the bandit in the blue car.

The difference in meaning between these two sentences is because in the first the phrase in the blue car modifies the policeman, whereas it modifies the bandit in the second.

2. Another important type of meaning that helps us to convey is in terms of the communicative or interactional function that we perform using language. The three most important communicative functions we perform using language and making statements, asking questions and making requests and grammar provides us with the most direct means of signalling these functions, as shown in the examples below.

Sheela has bought a new car.

Has Sheela bought a new car?

Who has bought a new car?

In the second sentence, a change in the order in which the subject Sheela and the auxiliary verb has occurs makes it a question, whereas in the third, the substitution of the question word who in the place of the subject Sheela makes it a question. Thus, we see that grammar also provides us with different means for asking different types of questions.

Please switch off the lights before you leave.

Turn right when you come to the intersection.

Take an asprin.

For functions like request, instructions and suggestions, we can use imperative sentences beginning with the imperative form of the verb as in the above usage.

3. We use language not only to convey factual information but also to convey our attitudes and feelings. Grammar often helps us to perform this attitudinal function.

Can I borrow your pen?

Could I borrow your pen?

The use of the past in the second sentence here makes it more polite than the first, which uses the present tense.

She always comes late.

She is always coming late.

The first sentence, which is in simple present tense (comes), is objective when compared with the second, which because of the use of the progressive aspect (is coming), appears more subjective implying criticism or disapproval.

4. When we communicate, we organize the information that we wish to convey in such a way that it is easy for the listener/the reader to understand our message. One of the principles we use is to begin with what is already known and then give the new information. It is this that helps us to choose between the two alternatives in the example below.

The famous author has written a sequel to his latest novel.

It has been highly praised by all the critics.

All the critics have praised it highly.

Of the two alternatives either can follow the first sentence. But the principle of beginning with what is already known (his latest novel in this sentence) will make us choose the first option instead of the second. This choice is between the passive and the active. Thus, we see that the grammatical feature of voice is related to how we organize information in our communication. Sometimes it is what we would like to emphasize in our message that decides our choice between the alternatives that grammar makes available.

A German scholar taught them Sanskrit.

It was a German scholar who taught them Sanskrit.

The difference between the two sentences is that in the second the emphasis is on a German scholar, which is here considered to be the most important bit of information conveyed.

Thus, grammar helps us to make subtle distinctions of meaning in terms of ideas, facts, thoughts and beliefs conveyed communicative functions performed like statements, questions and requests, attitudes and feelings conveyed like politeness, disapproval, etc, and information focus like indicating what is new information or what time of information is being emphasized.

Now that we have looked at the important concepts in grammar like grammatical units, chain and choice factors, grammatical structure and grammatical features and also the relationship between grammar and meaning, we can begin our study of English grammar.

THE SENTENCE AND TYPES OF SENTENCES

When we speak or write we use words. We generally use these words in groups, as:

Little jack Horner sat in a corner.

Hence, A group of words like this, which make a complete sense, is called a Sentence.

Kinds of Sentences

Sentences are of four kinds:

Those which make *statements or assertions*: as,

❑ Humpty dumpty sat on a wall.

Those which *ask questions*: as

❑ Where do you live?

Those which express *commands, requests, or entreaties*; as,

❑ Be quiet. Have mercy upon us.

Those which express *strong feelings*; as,

❑ How very cold the night is! What a shame!

✓ A sentence that makes a statement or assertion is called a *Declarative or Assertive Sentence*. Example: Sentence No-(1)

✓ A sentence that asks a question is called an *Interrogative Sentence*. Example: Sentence No-(2)

✓ A sentence that expresses a command or an entreaty is called an *Imperative Sentence*. Example- Sentence No-(3)

✓ A sentence that expresses strong feeling is called an *Exclamatory Sentence*. Example- Sentence No-(4)

Subject and Predicate

When we make a sentence:

We name some person or thing; and

Say something about that person or thing.

❑ In other words, we must have a *subject to speak* and *we must say or predicate something about the subject.*

Hence, every sentence has two parts:

The part which names the person or thing we are speaking about. This is called the subject of the sentence.

The part which tells something about the subject. *This is called the predicate of the sentence.*

The subject of a sentence usually comes first, but occasionally is put after the predicate; as

- ❑ Down went the royal George.
- ❑ Sweet are the uses of adversity.

In imperative sentences the subject is left out; as,

- ❑ Sit down. (Here the subject you is understood).
- ❑ Thank him. (Here too the subject you is understood).

Examine the group of words 'in a corner'. It makes sense, but not complete sense. Such group of words, which makes sense, but not completes sense, is called a phrase.

In the following sentences, the groups of words in italics are phrases:

The sun rises *in the east.*

Humpty dumpty *sat on a wall.*

There came a giant *to my door.*

It was *a sunset of great beauty.*

Examine the groups of words in italics in the following sentences:

He has *a chain of gold.*

He has *a chain which is made of gold.*

We recognise the first group of words as a phrase.

The second group of words, unlike the phrase of gold, contains a subject (which) and a predicate (is made of gold).

Such a group of words which forms a part of a sentence, and contains a subject and a predicate is called a clause.

In the following sentences, the groups of *words in italics are clauses*:

People *who pay their debts are trusted.*

We cannot start *while it is raining.*

I think that *you have made a mistake.*

EXERCISE

In the following sentences, separate the subject and the predicate. One has been done for you.

- ❑ The crackling of geese saved Rome.
    - ✓ The crackling of geese-Subject /Saved Rome-Predicate.
- ❑ The boy stood on the burning deck.
    - ✓
- ❑ Tubal Cain was a man of might.
    - ✓
- ❑ Stone walls do not a prison make.
    - ✓
- ❑ The singing of the birds delights us.
    - ✓
- ❑ Miss kitty was rude at the table one day.
    - ✓
- ❑ He has a good memory.
    - ✓
- ❑ Bad habits grow unconsciously.
    - ✓
- ❑ The earth revolves round the sun.
    - ✓
- ❑ Nature is the best physician.
    - ✓
- ❑ Edison invented the phonograph.
    - ✓
- ❑ The sea hath many thousand sands.
    - ✓
- ❑ We cannot pump the ocean dry.
    - ✓
- ❑ Borrowed garments never fit well.
    - ✓

- ❑ The early bird catches the worm.
  ✓ ....
- ❑ All matter is indestructible.
  ✓ ....
- ❑ Ascham taught Latin to Queen Elizabeth.
  ✓ ....
- ❑ We should profit by experience.
  ✓ ....
- ❑ All roads lead to Rome.
  ✓ ....
- ❑ A guilty conscience needs no excuse.
  ....

CHAPTER 2

THE PARTS OF SPEECH

Words are divided into different kinds or classes, called the **parts of speech**, according to their use; that is, according to the work they do in a sentence. The parts of speech are **eight** in number. They are as follows:

1. Noun	2. Adjective	3. Pronoun	4. Verb
5. Adverb	6. Preposition	7. Conjunction	8. Interjection

A **noun** is a word used as a name of a person, place or thing; as,

1. *Akbar* was a great *king*.   2. *Kolkata* is on the *Hooghly*.

3. The *rose* smells sweet.   4. The *sun* shines bright.

5. His *courage* won him *honour*.

> **Note** *The words in italics are **Nouns**.*

An **adjective** is a word used to add something to the meaning of a noun; as,

- ❏   He is a *brave* boy.
- ❏   There are *twenty* boys in this class.

The words in italics are Adjectives.

A **pronoun** is a word used instead of a noun; as,

John is absent, because *he* is ill.

The books are where you left *them*.

> **Note** *The words in italics are **Pronouns**.*

A **verb** is a word used to say something about some person, place or thing; as,

- ❏   The girl *wrote* a letter to her cousin.
- ❏   Mumbai *is* a busy city.
- ❏   Iron and copper *are* useful metals.

> **Note** *The words in italics are **Verbs**.*

An **adverb** is a word used to add something to the meaning of a verb, an adjective or another adverb; as,

- ❑ He worked the sum *quickly*.
- ❑ This flower is *very* beautiful.
- ❑ She pronounced the word *quite correctly*.

*A **preposition** is a word used with a noun or a pronoun to show how the person or thing denoted by the noun or pronoun stands in relation to something else' as,*

- ❑ There is a cow *in* the garden.
- ❑ The girl is fond *of* music.
- ❑ A fair little girl sat *under* a tree.

*A **conjunction** is a word used to join words or sentences together; as,*

- ❑ Rama *and* Hari are cousins.
- ❑ Two *and* two make four.
- ❑ I ran fast, *but* missed the train.

*An **interjection** is a word which expresses some sudden feeling; as,*

- ❑ *Hurrah!* We have won the game.
- ❑ *Alas!* She is dead.

As words are divided into different classes according to the work they do in sentences, it is clear that we cannot say to which part of speech a word belongs unless we see it used in a sentence.

They arrived *soon after*. Soon after-(Adverb)

They arrived *after* us. After-(Preposition)

They arrived *after* we had left. After-(Conjunction)

EXERCISE

Name the parts of speech of each italicised word in the following sentences, giving in each case your reason for the classification:

- ❑ *Still* waters run deep.
  ✓ ....

- ❑ He *still* lives in that house.
  ✓ ....

- ❑ *After* the storm comes the calm.
  ✓ ....

- ❑ The *aftereffects* of the drug are bad.
  ✓ ....

- ❑ The *up* train is late.
  ✓ ....

- ❑ It weighs *about* a pound.
  ✓ ....

- ❑ He told us all *about* the battle.
  ✓ ....

- ❑ He was only a yard *off* me.
  ✓ ....

- ❑ Suddenly one of the wheels came *off*,
  ✓ ....

- ❑ Mohammendans *fast* in the month of Ramzan.
  ✓ ....

- ❑ He kept the *fast* for a week.
  ✓ ....

- ❑ He is *on* the committee.
  ✓ ....

- ❑ Let us move *on*.
  ✓ ....

- ❑ Sit down and rest a *while*.
  ....

Chapter 3

NOUNS

A **noun** tells us what someone or something is called. For example, name of a person (John); a job title (Doctor); a name of a thing (radio);, name of a place (Delhi); name of a quality (courage) or the name of an action (laughter). Nouns are the names we give to people, things, places, etc., in order to identify them. Many nouns are used after a determiner, e.g., a boy, this house and often combine with other words to form a noun phrase e.g., the man next door; that big building, etc. nouns and noun phrases answer the questions: who or what. Nouns and noun phrases may be used as:

The subject of a verb:

   Our agent in Mumbai sent a message to us.

The direct object of a transitive verb:

   Our agent sent an urgent message.

The indirect object of a verb:

   Our agent sent a message to his manager.

The object of a preposition:

   I have seen it on the paper.

Used in apposition:

   Tarun, our agent sent a message.

Used when we speak directly to somebody:

   "Tarun, will you come tomorrow?"

Go through the table given below carefully. Write as many sentences as you can and underline the Nouns.

			a good teacher.
Jaya's	brother	is	a famous painter.
His	sister	was	an active politician
My	mother	will be	a dull worker.
Her	father		a rich lawyer.
Our	uncle		a popular doctor.
Their	aunt		a hard worker.
Your	nephew		a smooth runner.

26

SPOKEN ENGLISH

Read the table given below carefully. Make as many sentences as you can and underline the Nouns.

	Is	a bridge over the River Cauveri.
	was	a way out.
	was not	such a rumour.
	will be	a meeting.
Here	will not be	a conference.
There	has been	a great panic.
	has not been	a source of information.
	won't be	a call by the President.
	must be	a troop waiting.

Here all the sentences begin with the words, `Here' and `There'.

Kinds of Nouns

There are **five kinds of nouns: proper, common, collective, material and abstract**.

A **proper noun** is the name of a particular person, place or thing:

✓ Akbar, Raipur, the Taj Mahal.

A **common noun** is a name which is common to any and every person, place or thing of the same kind:

✓ Student, park, statue.

A **collective noun** denotes a number of persons or things grouped together as one complete whole:

✓ A *crowd* (a collection of people),

✓ A *flock* (a collection of sheep),

✓ A *fleet* (a collection of ships).

✓ A distinction is made between *a collective noun* and *a noun of multitude*. A collective noun denotes a collection and hence, a verb is singular; as,

✓ The committee consists of seven members.

✓ A *noun of multitude* denotes individuals of a group and hence, the verb is plural although the noun is singular; as,

✓ The committee (= the members composing the committee) quarrel among themselves.

A **material noun** denotes the matter or substance of which things are made, such as: Gold, silver, glass, cotton, steel, stone, etc.

An **abstract noun** is the name of some quality, state or action:

✓ Quality- Kindness, goodness, wisdom.

✓ State- Sickness, death, childhood, youth, slavery.

✓ Action- Laughter, movement, flight, revenge.

Countable and Uncountable Nouns

If a noun is countable:

We can use 'a' or 'an' in front of it: A book, an ant.

It has a plural and can be used in a question: how many?

You can use numbers :

- ✓ One stamp, two stamps.
- ✓ Uncountable nouns
- ✓ If a noun is uncountable:

We do not normally use 'a' or 'an' in front of it:

- ✓ Sugar is sweet.

It does not normally have a plural and it can be used in a question:

- ✓ How much?
- ❑ © We cannot normally use a number (one, two) in front of it.
- ❑ Give me some water.

A number of nouns are usually uncountable in English. A few common examples are: baggage, furniture, information, machinery, etc. eg.,

We brought new furniture for our house.

Give me some information on the topic.

We cannot use 'a' or a number before a mass (uncountable) noun. We cannot say a milk or two sugars. If we want to say how much milk or how much sugar, then we use a countable Noun+of (a bottle of milk, two kilos of sugar). The following are some examples of countable nouns in this pattern.

A glass of water	twenty liters of petrol	a tin of soup
A box of matches	a sheet of paper	a loaf of bread
A tube of toothpaste	a bar of chocolate	a jar of jam
A piece of wood	a cup of coffee	a slice of toast
A packet of washing powder	five meters of cable	ten grams of butter

Note *We can also use this pattern with a plural noun after 'of' e.g., a packet of chips, four kilos of potatoes.*

Collective Noun + Plural Verb

The following collective nouns must be followed by a plural verb; these nouns do not have plural forms:

Cattle, the clergy, the military, people, the police, swine, etc.

Some people are never satisfied.

The political/the military have surrounded the building.

Noun with A Plural Form + Singular Verb

The following nouns, though plural in form are always followed by a verb in the singular:

News: the news on T.V. is always depressing.

Games such as billiards, darts, dominoes:

Billiards is becoming more popular these days.

Names of cities such as Athens, Naples etc.

Athens has grown rapidly in the last decade.

Two Nouns Joined by 'And'

Nouns that commonly go together (bread and butter, lemon and oil, fish and chips, cheese and wine, etc) are used with verbs in the singular, when we think of them as a singular unit:

Fish and chips is a popular meal.

If we think of the items as separate we use a plural verb:

Fish and chips make a good meal.

EXERCISE

Complete the following sentences by filling in the blanks with 'a/an' or some. One has been done for you.

❑   *Example:* I ought to do ____ housework.

❑   *Answer*: I ought to do some housework.

Nitin is here for two nights, and he is looking for ____ accommodation.

I can't fit this book into ____ bag.

He is doing ____ research on radioactivity.

We are just about to set off on ____ long journey.

The people who camped in the field have left_____ rubbish.

This isn't right. Look, you've made____ mistake.

The scientists are doing _____ interesting experiment.

You need ____ luck to win at this game.

My room is quite empty. We need _____ furniture.

Can I get ___cup of coffee?

Answer					
(1.) an	(2.) a	(3.) some	(4.) a	(5.) Some	(6.) a
(7) an	(8.) some	(9.) some	(10.) A		

CHAPTER 4

PRONOUNS

A pronoun is a word that can be used in place of a noun or a noun phrase, as the word itself tells us: 'pro-noun'. For Example:

- ❏ Ravi arrived late. He had a headache.
- ❏ I wrote to my sister and told her what she should do.

Personal Pronouns

Personal pronouns refer to the speaker (first person), the person spoken to (second person), or the person, place or thing spoken about (third person. Personal pronouns must agree with nouns with the nouns in gender, number and person for which they stand:

Tarun is a naughty boy. He has been punished.

I brought a cake. It was fresh.

The apples are rotten. They have to be discarded.

- ❏ *When a pronoun stands for a collective noun. It must be singular in number*. If the collective noun is viewed as a single entity. If the collective noun conveys the idea of separate individuals composing the whole, then the plural number must be used:
  - ✓ The jury has given its verdict.
  - ✓ The jury were divided in their opinion.
- ❏ When two singular nouns joined by 'and' refer to the same person or thing, the pronoun should be singular; as:
  - ✓ The secretary and treasurer did not do his duty.

  But when two or more singular nouns joined by 'and' and refer to different persons the pronoun is in the plural:
  - ✓ Rita and Rahul have come. They are our artists.
  - ✓ *When two or more singular nouns joined by 'and' are preceded by 'each' or 'every' the pronoun must be singular:*Each policeman and each home guard was at his post.
- ❏ *When two or more singular nouns are joined by 'or' 'either… or' 'neither… nor', the pronoun must be singular.*

  Ravi or Rahul has lost his bag. Neither Ravi nor Rahul has done his work.

  But when a singular noun and a plural noun are joined by 'or' 'neither… nor' the pronoun is in the plural:

✓ Neither Ali nor his friends admitted their fault.

✓ Either the leader or his followers did not do their duty.

❑ *When a pronoun refers to more than one noun or pronoun of different persons, the pronoun agrees with the first person rather than with the second or third person, and it agrees with the second rather than with the third; as*

✓ He and I completed our work.

✓ You and he have wasted your time.

❑ *With transitive verbs, the choice between the subjects form and the object form of a pronoun depends on the context and the meaning.*

✓ You love him as much as I.

✓ She loves you more than me.

Reflexive and Emphasising Pronouns

Reflexive and emphasising pronouns are: Myself, yourself, himself, herself, itself, ourselves, yourselves and themselves.

Used as reflexive pronouns myself, yourself etc are used as objects of a verb when the action of the verb returns to the doer. That is, in such a situation the subject and the object refer to the same person or thing: as,

❑ They hurt themselves.

❑ He shot himself.

Used as emphasising pronouns myself, yourself etc are used to emphasise a noun or a pronoun ; as,

❑ You yourself can best explain.

❑ She herself can do it.

Relative Pronouns

The pronouns who, which, that, what, etc., which join two sentences and relate to nouns which have gone before are called Relative Pronouns. The noun to which a relative pronoun refers is called its Antecedent.

❑ This is the boy who gave me a pen.

✓ In this sentence, boy is the antecedent of the Relative pronoun 'who'.

The following are the forms of the relative pronouns.

Nominative	Possessive	Objective
Who	Whose	Whom
Which	Of which	Which
That	Of that	That
What	Of what	What

Uses of Relative Pronouns

The relative pronoun always agrees with its Antecedent in number, gender and person.

WHO is used for persons only; as:

- ✓ Blessed is he who works hard.
- ✓ God helps those who help themselves.

WHICH is used for animals and for things without life; as:

- ✓ He found the dog which was lost.
- ✓ This is the pen which I gave you yesterday.

THAT is used for persons, animals and things; as:

- ✓ Uneasy lies the head that wears the crown.
- ✓ He that is down need fear no fall.

WHAT is used for things only. Its antecedent is always understood; as:

- ✓ I say what I mean.
- ✓ Attend to what he says.

Omission of the Relative Pronoun and its Antecedent

The relative pronoun in the objective case is generally omitted; as:

- ✓ I am the monarch of all (that) I survey.
- ✓ This is the village (that) we live in.

Sometimes the antecedent of a relative pronoun is omitted ; as:

Whom the gods love, die young.

Who laughs last laughs best.

EXERCISE

Choose the correct word from each bracket and complete the sentence.

- ❑ We scored as many goals as (they, them).
- ❑ Whom can I trust, if not (she, her).
- ❑ I am one year older than (he, him).
- ❑ I am richer than (they, them).
- ❑ He is as good a student as (she, her)
- ❑ The hotel (which, what) we stayed at last summer is now closed.
- ❑ The boy (who, whom) fell off his bicycle has hurt his leg.
- ❑ I have not seen the boy (whose, whom) suitcase was stolen.
- ❑ Kalidasa was a great poet (who, that) wrote interesting plays.
- ❑ Rekha is the maid (who, whom) I have employed.

Join together each of the following pairs of sentences by means of a relative pronoun:

- ❑ Here is the book. I told you about it.
- ❑ Did you receive the parcel? I sent the parcel yesterday.
- ❑ Ramesh tells lies. He deserves to be punished.
- ❑ Here is the doctor. The doctor cured me of fever.
- ❑ This is the man. We were saved through his courage.
- ❑ Show me the road. The road leads to the airport.
- ❑ The boy won the first prize. You see him sitting there.
- ❑ They heard some news. The news astonished them.
- ❑ She spoke to the victim. The victim's arm was in a sling.
- ❑ The conference was a success. It was held in Pune.

CHAPTER 5

VERBS

A *Verb* is the most important word in a sentence. *Verbs* are mostly called as the *action words*. This tells us what a person does or what the work or action is being done. For example:

(1.) He <u>writes</u>.
(2.) She <u>sings</u>.
(3.) The thief <u>was</u> <u>arrested</u>.
(4.) What a person he <u>is</u>!
(5.) He <u>is</u> an honest man.
(6.) What a person he <u>has been</u>!
(7.) He <u>has</u> many friends.

Verbs are of two kinds: Transitive Verbs and Intransitive Verbs.

Transitive Verbs: In a sentence or syntax, a transitive verb is a verb that requires one or more objects to complete its sense. The term is used in contrast to the intransitive verbs, which do not have objects.

Example: Please **bring** me a glass of water.

Basically, Transitive Verb is a verb that must be followed by a direct object. The following chart shows a number of Transitive Verbs and the Sentences formed by them.

bring	Please <u>bring</u> me a glass of water.	buy	Do not <u>buy</u> chocolates from that shop.
cost	My coat <u>costs</u> a lot of money.	get	My children <u>get</u> good grades in school.
give	Our family <u>gives</u> gifts at Christmas.	leave	I <u>leave</u> home at 8:00 in the morning.
lend	Could you please <u>lend</u> me five dollars?	make	Did you <u>make</u> coffee this morning?
offer	My boss <u>offered</u> me a new job.	owe	I <u>owe</u> you ten rupees.
pass	All the students <u>passed</u> the test.	pay	Don't <u>forget</u> to pay the phone bill.
play	Susan <u>loves</u> playing the piano.	promise	She <u>promised</u> me she would come to the party.

read	They <u>read</u> the newspaper every day.	refuse	The custom officers <u>refused</u> to let me enter the country.
send	My girlfriend <u>sends</u> me an e-mail message every day.	show	My neighbour <u>showed</u> me her garden yesterday.
sing	Janet sings songs at the church every Sunday night.	take	Travellers take planes or trains to their destinations.
teach	Our parents teach us to be kind.	tell	The author wrote a good story.

Intransitive Verbs: In a sentence or syntax, an intransitive verb is a verb that does not require one or more objects to complete its sense. The term is used in contrast to the transitive verbs, which do have objects.

Verbs make tenses, and as such, they have three forms:

(Present)	(Past)	(Past Participle)
Walk	Walked	Walked
Want	Wanted	Wanted

Note

Such verbs are called regular verbs. There are irregular verbs also like:

I	II	III
Go	went	gone
Be (is am are)	was were	been
Buy	bought	bought
Become	became	become
Beat	beat	beaten (pronounced as <u>bat</u>)

I	II	III
Telecast	telecast	telecast
Broadcast	broadcast	broadcast
Cost	cost	cost
Cut	cut	cut
Shut	shut	shut
Put	put	put
Read	read	read
		(pronounced as red)

13.4 *The three forms of verbs do not exactly refer to the three tenses:*

I	II	III
Go	went	gone

He will go. (Present Tense)

He went (Past Tense)

He will go. (Future Tense)

He has gone (Past Participle in perfect tenses)

Note

To make future tense we use shall/ will with first form of verb.
Has, have, had are always used with the past participle or third form of verb to make perfect tenses.

EXERCISE

Choose suitable verbs from the following to complete the sentences given below:

Are, is, am, has, have, had, was

(1.) This bank _____ four branches in the city.

(2.) These _____ not a drop of water in the glass.

(3.) Students of this section _____ not serious in their studies.

(4.) _____ these cars not sleek and beautiful?

(5.) He _____ not at home.

(6.) It _____ midnight when he came home.

(7.) Last winter it _____ very cold Ooty.

(8.) I _____ many book. You can take a few.

(9.) He _____ no money he died in twenty.

(10.) _____ you any money.

(11.) I _____ not dishonest.

Answers					
(1.) has	(2.) is	(3.) are	(4.) are	(5.) is	(6.) was
(7.) was	(8.) have	(9.) had	(10.) have	(11.) am	

Using **tense** and **verbs,** complete the conversation between two friends:

(1.) Ved: Hello Rohit! I'm _____ you after a long time. We _____ since long. _____ we?

(2.) Rohit: Yes, it _____ long since we saw each other.

(3.) Ved: Where _____ you _____?

(4.) Rohit: Oh! My boss _____ me to Mumbai on some errand.

(5.) I _____ to go but since.

(6.) I _____ a job, I _____.

(7.) Ved: In which office _____ you work?

(8.) __ it the old one?

(9.) Rohit: No, I do not work there now. I _____ my forever boss but then this boss _____ me. Same unpleasant situation.

(10.) Ved: Why ___ it so?

(11.) Rohit: _____usually late. Others _____ also at times late, but he always scolds and humiliates me because he _____me.

(12.) Ved: That ____rather sad. Why can't you __punctual?

(13.) Rohit: I _____since long but something or the other_____. One day he _____very angry. He _____quite a temper, you know. At that time, I _____so ashamed. After all, he _____ an office and besides, he _____very sincere.

(14.) Ved: I must _____ what ____ going on ___bad as you _____it, _____on since long, I _____ you _____another job, or else _____ your ways, otherwise your boss _____you.

(15.) Rohit: He is not that kind, believe me. As I told you, just now that he sent me to Mumbai and I did good work there. When I _____ back, I reported to him as to what _____ there in the meetings. Who _____, who _____ not, what _____ and what _____ the end result.

(16.) Ved: Was your boss_____?

(17.) Rohit: I dare say, yes. He _____me many questions. He asked me how many people_____, what _____ they actually _____ and for how long a particular, Mr. Sinha _____the various aspects of the project?

(18.) Ved: _____glad to hear it. _____ he _____ you there again?

(19.) Rohit: No, he _____ me there again, maybe, I _____ to some other place.

(20.) Ved: When ___that?

(21.) Rohit: After I _____my Mumbai project report to him. I _____it by now, but other works also _____up.

(22.) Ved: Good luck to you. When _____ we _____ again?

(23.) Rohit: Soon. _____upon you.

Answers

(1). Seeing, haven't met, Have
(2.) has been
(3). Have, been
(4). Sent
(5). Didn't want
(6). Do, had to go
(7). Do,
(8). Is
(9). Didn't like, Doesn't like
(10). Is,
(11). I'm, are, doesn't like
(12). Is, be
(13). Have been, happens, has, felt, runs, is
(14). Say, is, is, have said, has been going, suggest, find, change, will fire
(15). Is, told, sent, came, did, was discussed, was
(16). Pleased
(17). Asked, had come, were, discussing, had been discussing,
(18). I'm, will, send
(19). Won't send, will be going
(20). Is
(21). Have submitted, will have prepared
(22). Do, meet
(23). I'll call Answ

Chapter 6

ADJECTIVES

Adjectives literally means 'added to.' A word which adds details to the noun (or the pronoun) or describes it is called an adjective; as,

- ✓ She has a **pretty** dress.
- ✓ The table is **large**.

Adjectives are used ether attributively or predicatively. We say that an adjective is used attributively, when it is placed before a noun, such as:

- ✓ The **brave** soldier was honoured.
- ✓ It is a **bright** day.

When an adjective is used after the verb as a part of the predicate, it is said t be used predicatively:

- ✓ The soldier was **brave**.
- ✓ The day is **bright**.

A few adjectives such as old, late and heavy can take a different meaning when they are used attributively as:

Note
- ✓ Simon peter is an **old** friend.
- ✓ My late grandfather was a **miner**.

All the words in Bold are Adjectives or Describing Words.

Kinds of Adjectives

Adjectives may be divided into the following classes:

(1.) **Adjectives of Quality** answer the question: of what kind? They show the kind of quality of a person or thing; as,

- ❑ He is a *clever* boy.
- ❑ *Indian* goods are sold abroad.
  - ✓ Adjectives formed from proper nouns (e.g., *Indian* goods, *French* perfumes, *English* language, etc.) are sometimes called Proper Adjectives. They are generally classed with adjectives of Quality.

(2.) Adjectives of Quantity

- ❑ Adjectives of quantity answer the question, how much? They show how much of a thing is meant; as,

- ✓ He ate *some* bread.
- ✓ We have had *enough* exercise.

(3.) **Adjectives of Number** answer the question, how many, or in what order. They show how many persons or things are meant, or in what order a person or thing stands; as,

- ✓ Take *some* ripe bananas.
- ✓ *Few* boys want to take risks.

(4.) **Demonstrative Adjectives** answer the question, 'which'? They point out which person or thing is meant; as,

- ✓ Those girls must be rewarded.
- ✓ This boy is brave.

(5.) **Interrogative Adjectives**

- ❏ Interrogative adjectives are used with nouns to ask question; as,
  - ✓ Whose shirt is this?
  - ✓ Which road leads to the town?

(6.) **Emphasising Adjectives**

- ❏ Emphasizing adjectives are own and very; as,
  - ✓ I saw it with my own eyes.
  - ✓ This is the very man who killed the tiger.

(7.) **Exclamatory Adjectives**

- ❏ What is sometimes used as an exclamatory adjective; as,
  - ✓ What an idea! What luck!
  - ✓ What a piece of work man is!

(8.) **Adjectives Used as Nouns**

- ❏ Adjectives are sometimes used as nouns: as,
  Certain adjectives, preceded by the, can be used as nouns in the plural sense. They denote a class of persons:
  - ✓ Blessed are the meek
  - ✓ The rich do not care for the poor.
- ❏ *Some adjectives, preceded by the, denote some abstract quality:*
  - ✓ The future is unknown to us.
  - ✓ He admires the good.
- ❏ *Some adjectives actually become nouns and can be used both in the singular and in the plural:*
  - ✓ Junior, juniors; senior, seniors; Italian, Italians; superior, superiors; elder, elders; mortals; inferior, inferiors; Indian, Indians, etc.
- ❏ *In certain phrases and idioms, the adjectives are used as nouns:*
  - ✓ I shall see you before long.

EXERCISE

Go through the table carefully and make as many sentences as you can. Also underline all the adjectives in the following sentences.

		authentic flags.
		street dogs.
		modern houses.
		pet birds.
		rough copies.
		intelligent boys.
		house plants.
		rainy coats.
		weather charts.
These	are	race horses.
Those	were	steel chairs.
		regular beggars.
		green trees.
		old pants.
		new maps.
		Indian cows.
		mild animals.
		text books.
		working girls.
		new benches.
		half shirts.
		right keys.
		table fans.
		cheap mobiles.
		costly computers.

Note

For Example: ***These are authentic flags.***
                                      These are street dogs.
                                       Those are authentic flags.
                                       Those are street dogs.

Form as many sentences as you can and underline the adjectives. Also specify the kind of adjective in each case.

Is was	it that	not a/the	very hot day? wintery night? Sunday afternoon? month of April? a sunny day? cloudy sky? foggy weather? a dense forest? a beautiful garden? a cool evening? a delicious dish? a rough way? a mammoth gathering? the public opinion? the general rule?	?

Note *All the sentences formed from the above table end with Question Marks and are Negative Sentences.*

Form as many sentences as you can from the table given below, then identify and underline the adjectives. Also specify the kind of adjective in each case.

There		five flags. big houses. small birds. plenty of boys. tall plants. innumerable coats. black horses. uncomfortable chairs. huge trees. only blue pants.

		two world maps.
	are	few old cows.
	were	some religious books.
		a whole lot of benches.
		bright shirts.
		no keys here.

Note *All the sentences formed from the above table are plural in number and are both in Present and Past Tenses.*

Form as many sentences as you can from the table below, then underline the adjectives. Also specify the kind of adjective in each case.

			authentic flags.
			street dogs.
These	are	not	modern houses.
Those	were		rough copies.
			intelligent boys.
			weather charts.
			race horses.
			wild animals.
			working girls.
			cheap mobiles.
			costly computers.

Note *All the sentences formed from the above table are plural in number and are negative in character.*

CHAPTER 2

ADVERBS

The word, Adverb suggests the idea of adding to the meaning of a verb. Adverbs tell us something about the action in a sentence by modifying a verb, an adjective, an adverb, a prepositional phrase, a sentence or a conjunction: as,

Verb	:	She sang well.
Adjective	:	He was awfully hungry.
Other adverb	:	We will come very soon.
Prepositional phrase	:	You are entirely in the wrong.
Complete sentence	:	Fortunately, I won the first prize.
Conjunction	:	He comes here only when my father is present.

The following sentences show how adverbs affect the meaning of a sentence. Compare:

Harry has left.   Harry has *just* left.

I have finished work.   I have *nearly* finished work.

Kinds of Adverb

There are three kinds of Adverbs: Simple, Interrogative, and Relative.

Simple Adverbs

Simple adverbs modify words. They can be divided into the following groups:

(1.) *Adverbs of Time* (which show when): now, then, before, soon, tomorrow, already etc:
   - ✓ The president is now in his office.
   - ✓ I have spoken to the principal already.

(2.) *Adverbs of Place* (which show where): here, there, everywhere, in, out, etc:
   - ✓ He looked for me everywhere.
   - ✓ He had come here.

(3.) *Adverbs of Manner* (which show how or in what manner): well, badly, thus, so, etc.
   - ✓ Slowly and sadly we laid him down.

(4.) Adverbs of frequency (which show how often): once, twice sometimes, seldom, etc.
   - ✓ I have often made mistakes. He has already met me twice.

(5.) *Adverbs of Degree or Quantity (*which show how much or to what extent or in what degree) : very, much, almost, wholly, quite, extent, rather, etc:

- ✓ The water is very cold.
- ✓ The weather is very pleasant.
- ✓ He is altogether mistaken.

(6.) *Adverbs of Reason* (therefore, likewise, etc.):

- ✓ She is hence absent from school.
- ✓ He was, therefore, put in detention.

(7.) *Adverbs of Affirmation or Negation* (yes, certainly, surely, no, never, etc):

- ✓ I shall certainly attend the meeting.
- ✓ He will never come.

Interrogative Adverbs

These adverbs are used in asking questions; as,

Time	:	When will you come again?
Place	:	Where are you going?
Manner	:	How do you intend helping me?
Number or frequency	:	How many people were present?
Degree, extent or quantity	:	How deep is the well?
Reason	:	Why did you do this?

Relative Adverbs

Relative adverbs modify some word in a clause; they also connect the clause in which they occur with the rest of the sentence. The antecedent noun to which they relate may be either omitted or expressed.

- ❑ The antecedent expressed : as,
  - ✓ This is the school where I studied.
  - ✓ I do not know the time when it rained.
- ❑ The antecedent omitted; as,
  - ✓ This is where (the place in which) we met earlier.
  - ✓ I did not know when (the time by which) he had come.

Uses of Some Adverbs

TOO, VERY

- ❑ The adverb 'too' means excess of some kind or more than enough. It should not be used in place of very or much; as,
  - ✓ This news is too good to be true.
  - ✓ We shall be too late for the show.

- ✓ 'Very' merely means much:
- ✓ It is very hot today. He is very kind.

MUCH, VERY

❑ 'Much' is used before past participles. 'Very' before present participles
- ✓ I was much disturbed by his behaviour.
- ✓ His behaviour is very annoying even now.

❑ 'Much' is used with adjectives and adverbs in the comparative degree. 'Very' is used in the positive degree:
- ✓ I feel much better today.
- ✓ He walked very slowly.

BEFORE, AGO, SINCE

❑ 'Before' as an adverb means formerly; as,
- ✓ He reached here an hour before.
- ✓ He has been to Shimla before.

❑ 'Ago' denotes a period of time from the present dating backwards. 'Since' recons from a point of time in the past up to the present:
- ✓ His father died three years ago.
- ✓ He has not met me before.
- ✓ I have not seen him since last Christmas.

FAIRLY, RATHER

❑ Both mean moderately. 'Fairly' is mainly used with favourable adjectives and adverbs while 'rather' is used with unfavourable adjectives and adverbs.
- ✓ She is fairly rich, but her aunt is rather poor.
- ✓ I did fairly well in the examination, but my friend did rather badly.

EXERCISE

Fill in the blanks with the suitable words from the brackets:

1. He spoke loud _____ to be heard. (much, enough).
2. It is _____ late, but not _____ late to catch the train. (too, very)
3. She waited for us _____ impatiently. (very, much)
4. Fruit is _____ cheap today, but is _____ dear for me to buy any. (too, very)
5. This magazine is _____ heavy, but that one is _____ light. (fairly, rather)
6. This news is _____ good to be true (very, too)
7. It is _____ hot to go outside. (very, much)
8. Our school closed a fortnight _____ (since, ago)
9. She has been absent from school _____ last Monday. (since, ago)
10. The patient is _____ better today. (too, much)

Answers				
(1.) Enough	(2.) Very/too	(3.) Very	(4.) Very/too	(5.) Rather, fairly
(6.) Too	(7.) Very	(8.) Ago	(9.) Since	(10.) Much

Insert the words in brackets at suitable places:

1. We lost the match. (nearly)
2. He makes a mistake. (rarely)
3. He did well in the examination. (fairly)
4. The pupils have completed the class work. (almost)
5. Has her brother been a school master? (always)
6. His father had to work hard for his living. (never)
7. I am late for my lectures. (often)
8. He was tall to reach the shelf. (enough)
9. Does he make mistakes? (usually)
10. I was able to hear what they said. (hardly)
11. The teacher has marked these papers. (just)
12. He has travelled by train. (never)
13. We deceive ourselves. (sometimes)
14. I know her well. (quite)
15. He makes a mistake. (rarely)

CHAPTER 8

PREPOSITIONS AND THEIR USAGE

A preposition is a word usually placed before a noun or pronoun to show its relation to 'some other word' in a sentence as:

1. There is a pen on the book.
2. She is fond of music.
3. Jane jumped into the river.

The above words in italics are prepositions.

Usage of Some Common Prepositions

AT, IN, ON

- ❑ *Usage of AT*
  - ✓ Hope to see you *at* 10 o' clock at the dining table.
  - ✓ They began their journey *at* sunset.
- ❑ *Usage of IN*
  - ✓ *In* the next few days, I will be leaving from Mumbai.
  - ✓ *In* the summer holidays, I may visit my uncle's house at Jaipur.
  - ✓ *In* July, Sourav's school will reopen after the summer vacations.
  - ✓ *In* the 19th century, many milestones were achieved in Medical Science.
  - ✓ Make sure you are at the station *in* time for the train.
- ❑ *Usage of ON*
  - ✓ The 7.30 train started *on* time.
  - ✓ *On* arriving late for the meeting, he rushed into the room.
  - ✓ *On* hearing the sad news, she fainted on the floor.

AT, IN and ON: In Respect of Place

1. Someone is knocking at the door.
2. The car was waiting at the gate.

1. He lives in Moga in Punjab.

2. He works in Kolkata in India.

3. He lives at Panjim in Goa.

1. Look at the picture on the wall.

2. Spread the carpet on the floor.

3. Delhi is on the Yamuna.

4. My shop is right on the main road.

ON, UPON

- ❏ She sat *on* a sofa.
- ❏ The tiger pounced *upon* the deer.

IN, INTO

- ❏ The fish is *in* the water.
- ❏ Mohan jumped *into* the swimming pool.

IN, WITHIN

- ❏ I will return *in* a month. (at the close of)
- ❏ I will return *within* a month. (in less than)

IN, AFTER

- ❏ They shall finish the construction *in* a week.
- ❏ He reached Mumbai *after* two days.

FOR, SINCE, AGO

- ❏ I stayed in Delhi *for* a week.
- ❏ Please wait *for* five minutes.
- ❏ I have lived here *since* 1975.
- ❏ I haven't met her *since* September.
- ❏ I joined the school nine years *ago*.
- ❏ We came to your house two months *ago*.

BETWEEN, AMONG

- ❏ Divide the bananas *between* the two children.
- ❏ A dispute arose *between* the landlord and the tenant.

- ❏ The four sisters quarrelled *among* themselves.
- ❏ There is said to be an understanding *among* the thieves.

BESIDE, BESIDES

❑ They sat *beside* him.

❑ *Besides* being fined, they were imprisoned.

TILL/UNTIL, BY

❑ He sat in the shop *till/until* closing time.

❑ I'll be working in the office *till/until* next June.

❑ I get up *by* 6 o'clock.

❑ Please return my book *by* Monday.

BY, WITH

❑ She stood *by* her father.

❑ He sat *by* himself.

❑ She eats *with* me, talks *with* me and walks *with* me.

❑ *With* all her faults, I love her.

BEFORE, FOR

❑ He shall be there *before* 8 o'clock.

❑ We shall not be there *before* 4 o' clock.

❑ I have not seen her *for* a long time.

❑ He has been going to the gym *for* a week.

ABOVE, OVER

❑ The aeroplane flew *above* the clouds.

❑ High *above* us an eagle was hovering.

❑ The bridge *over* the river is long.

❑ The aeroplane flew *over* the town.

EXERCISE

Use appropriate preposition/s, and fill in the blanks describing a day alone at home.

After having read the newspaper, I decided to have lunch ___ *McDonald's*. It is only a ten-minute walk _____my house. Before I left, I gave some milk ____the cat.____McDonald's, I had a hearty meal. In addition to the delicious hamburger, I also had a chocolate ice cream. The meal was delicious as I sipped coke _____the bites. _____ the crowd at the McDonald's, there were many foreigners also. I would have sat _____ longer but had __ leave immediately after my meal because of the heavy crowd. As I stood ____ and walked ____ of the restaurant, I realised that it was very hot _____. I wanted to reach home quickly but _____ paid a brief visit to a bookstore and bought a novel. After all, I had to plan the rest of the day alone. As soon as I reached home, I switched ___the air conditioner and went to sleep at once. _____ I slept, the cat kept ___making noises because perhaps, it had seen a mouse__ the kitchen. I read the novel for some time and then started to cook food as I had no mood to go out. I ate my dinner around 9 pm, watched TV____late and then fed the cat before going __ sleep. I woke __only when my family came early __the morning.

Choose a suitable word from the ones given in brackets and complete the sentence in each case.

1. The children sat (on/upon) the ground.
2. One should live (in/within) one's means.
3. We must trust (in/on) our close friends.
4. The train is (after/behind) time.
5. Three thieves quarrelled (between/among) themselves.
6. He arrived (by/with) all his belongings.
7. She was (in/at) Kolkata last night.
8. She has been ill (since/for) last night.
9. We will return (in/on) an hour.
10. We returned from the picnic (after/since) three days.

CONJUNCTION

A conjunction is a word which joins two words or clauses together; as,

- ❑   I eat bread *and* butter.
- ❑   Two *and* two makes four.

Types of Conjunctions

Correlative Conjunctions

Conjunctions which are used in pairs are called correlative conjunctions; as,

1.   Either.... or: Either he is a fool or he is a rogue.
2.   Neither....nor: Neither a borrower nor a lender be.
3.   Both... and: He was both praised and rewarded.
4.   Not only .... but also: Not only is he foolish, but also obstinate.
5.   Whether... or: I do not care whether you eat or not.

Coordinating Conjunctions

These join together words, phrases or clauses of equal rank. They are of four kinds:

Cumulative Conjunctions: An additive conjunction merely adds one statement to another. It doesn't express ideas, such as contrast, choice or inference. Examples are: And, also, too, as well as, both...and, not only...but also...

- ✓   Pay your taxes and live in peace.
- ✓   He is both a teacher and a preacher.

Alternative Conjunctions: These express an alternative or a choice between two statements.

- ✓   She must weep or she will die.
- ✓   I have neither a pen nor a pencil.

Subordinating Conjunctions

Subordinating conjunctions may be classified according to their meanings, as follows:

Time: The train arrived after the signal had been lowered.

                        The man had died before the doctor arrived.

Cause and Reason:	I will give up my claim since you insist on it.
	Let us go to bed as it is midnight.
Concession or Contrast:	Although he is poor he is honest.
	You cannot deceive him, however you may try.

Underline the conjunctions used in this letter describing your visit to Mussoorie at your friend's place.

Dear Rahul,

How are you? It's been a long time that I didn't hear from you. How's life and how are Mona and your little one, Preeti? Hope they are all doing fine and hope Anty is also at the best of her health and mind. Do you remember Lata, my best friend? We all had such fun in her marriage at Delhi, long time back and teased her badly that she would lead a Polar Bear's life as she was getting married to an Engineer settled in Mussoorie!

I visited her last summer as she had called me a number of times and insisted that I visit her place at least once even if it was a short stay.

This time I thought, I should accept her invitation and plan a short trip to Mussorie. Moreover, I was sick and tired of my routine and hectic life at Delhi as well as desperately wanted a break and relief from the scorching heat and dust of Delhi during May and June which is almost killing. Moreover, the climate of Mussoorie is best during these months, though it is the peak tourist season and is very crowed at this time of the year by tourists from across the globe. However, I didn't have to worry about all this as Lata had written a lot about her big flat, etc. I have a relative in Mt. Abu too, who keeps calling me now and then inviting me to come over, but I decided to visit Lata, instead. Its been really long that I had seen her and we were such bosom friends all through our schooling in Delhi.

I booked my ticket in the tourist bus that started from ISBT, Old Delhi, stopped at a place for an hour for lunch and then straightaway stopped at Dehradun for some refreshments. Here, we saw the beautiful and famous waterfall called the *Sahastradhara* near Dehradun. We took a lot of photographs but couldn't take a shower in the Blessed Sulphur Springs of the Waterfall due to lack of time and the anxiety to reach Mussoorie and meet my friend after 10 years. I found the city of Dehradun quite noisy, populated and as hot as Delhi.

However, as we travelled further and climbed up several mountains on our way, the air began to get cooler and cooler. By the time, I reached the well-known Mall Road of Mussoorie, it had become really pleasant, cool and nice – a great change and relief from the heat of Delhi. Finally, I reached my friend's flat which was a walking distance from the noisy Mall Road full of tourists from all over India as May and June are generally the busiest months in hill stations. As I reached, I found my friend, Lata anxiously waiting for me at the entrance. We hugged each other warmly as her cute little five-year old daughter stared at us totally bewildered.

Then, of course as I handed over a number of chocolates and a gift pack. She gave me a broad smile and ran inside the house crying aloud calling her father as it was a Sunday and everyone was at home. Her mother called her back to formally introduce her, but she was too overwhelmed to receive a gift and was in a hurry to open it as soon as possible. She tore open the gift wrap and gave out almost a yell to lo and behold—a beautiful red coloured remote control car! Lata told me later that 'Red' was her favourite colour and she was crazy of all sorts of cars.

After a formal introduction with Lata's hubby, whom I had just met once during their marriage, almost 10 years back was equally surprised and delighted to see me. Actually, Lata had not told him anything about my visit, and it was indeed a pleasant surprise for him. Later, we all settled for coffee and of course, a long chat. Thanks to the helpful maid that Lata had kept mainly for her five-year-old daughter as she took my luggage into the room, prepared hot water for my bath and also cooked a delicious meal for all of us which included absolutely mouthwatering Vegetable Fried Rice made from the exclusive and aromatic Basmati Rice of Dehradun and Mattar Paneer, along with hot and crisp Pappad and Boondi Raita.

The next morning by about 11 am or so, me and friend along with her little angel set out for the Famous Kempty Falls of Mussoorie and this time we were all equipped to take a shower in the fall as many tourists do. We thoroughly enjoyed and the little one was jumping and hopping all around with immense joy and excitement. We were later joined by Lata's husband, Raghu at lunch in the Mall Road, as he was a C.P.W.D Engineer posted there. He took a half day leave, we had a sumptuous lunch at a Chinese Restaurant and then became busy strolling and shopping in the Mall which is considered to be the favourite pastime of almost all the tourists who come here.

The next day Lata and her husband took me to the famous temple nearby and from there we had a pony ride again to the Mall Road. Lata's daughter was thrilled by all this as she danced around like a little fairy dressed a beautiful pink fock! Finally, we ended our day with a one-hour ride on the Electric Ropeway Trolley over the Gun Hill—famous and historic from the time of the Britishers—a tour all over Mussoorie. I was indeed scared all through the ride as I watched breathlessly the altitude at which the trolley car moved, but to my great astonishment, the height and the ride both didn't scare the little one a bit. She was untiringly enthusiastic and eager, singing and dancing all through the journey, high up in the air, along with the sailing clouds, above the mountain peaks and rooftops as if she was all set to visit a fairyland that she has always dreamt of.

Three cool days passed by like anything and the nights were cooler. There was a fireplace at one of the corners of the huge drawing room in my friend's house with comfortable sofas, an exotic teakwood centre table with wood carvings and glass on the top of it, antique pieces of souvenirs and decorative items, some landscape paintings created by my friend, Lata as it was her hobby right from her school days. There were room heaters in both the bedrooms. Evenings and nights were really windy and chilly, but mornings and afternoons were beautiful and pleasant.

I never realised how four days had passed and I was at the end of my wonderful and memorable trip. I thoroughly enjoyed my brief stay at Mussoorie and at times, almost became a child with Lata's daughter, Pari.

I am really looking forward to visit them again and this time with my husband and son, who is three years younger to Pari. I wonder if Pari still remembers me!

Yours affectionately

Radha

EXERCISE

Choose the suitable conjunctions from the following and fill in the blanks.

Neither – nor, by. till, during, either – or, or else, even – though, despite, although, both at the end, Though – yet, while, unless, despite, in the end.

1. _____ you _____ your brother is guilty.
2. Wait here _____ I came back.
3. _____ you work hard you'll not pass the examination.
4. _____ he is poor _____ he is honest.
5. Behave yourself _____ I'll ask you leave the room.
6. You shouldn't buy any of these shirts. _____ black _____ white.
7. _____ of the candidates succeeded because _____ were rejected by the interview board.
8. _____ the weather was rainy, I went out for a walk.
9. _____ he doesn't speak French, he should still go to Paris.
10. _____ being sick, she went to take the examination.
11. He fell asleep _____ seeing the film.
12. My father was back _____ the time I reached home.
13. I won the argument _____.
14. He became nervous _____ the exam.
15. I was quite tired _____ of the day

Answers				
(1.) Either/or	(2.) Till/until	(3.) Unless	(4.) Though/yet	(5.) Or else
(6.) Neither/nor	(7.) Neither/ both	(8.) Even though	(9.) Although	(10.) Despite
(11.) While	(12.) By	(13.) In the end	(14.) During	(15.) At the end.

Fill in the blanks with appropriate conjunctions.

1. She was ___ill___ she could not study.
2. Strike _____ the iron___ is hot.
3. _____ she is poor, ___ she is honest.
4. _____ he tells the truth, he will be spared.
5. I brought it _____ I needed it.
6. Many strange things have happened ___ they came here.
7. Take heed _____ you fall.

8. Please write____ she dictates.
9. Make hay___ the sun shines.
10. Rita is pretty ____ not proud.

INTERJECTION

An interjection is a word which expresses some sudden feeling or emotion. A short utterance that usually expresses emotion and is capable of standing alone is called an Interjection. Interjections are generally considered as one of the traditional parts of speech.

In writing, an interjection, it is typically followed by an exclamation point. For Example:

Examine the following sentences:

Hello! What are you doing here?

Alas! He is dead.

Hurrah! We have won the game.

Ah! Have they gone?

Oh! I got such a fright.

Hush! Don't make a noise.

Hello! Alas! Hurrah! Ah! Etc. They are called Interjections.

All the underlined words written above are Interjections.

Basically, they are used to express some sudden feeling or emotion. It will be noticed that they are not grammatically related to the other words in a sentence.

An Interjection may express:

Joy; as Hurrah! Huzza!

Grief; as, Alas!

Surprise; as, Ha! What!

Approval; as, Bravo!

Certain groups of words are also used to express some sudden feeling or emotion; as,

Ah me! For shame! Well done! Good gracious!

> **Note**
>
> *Basically, Interjections express the extreme feelings or emotions while speaking or writing Good English and they are used when one expresses extreme joy, sadness, fear, surprise, anxiety, etc.*

EXERCISE

Underline the Interjections in the sentences given below. The first one has been done for you.

1. Hey! You left me behind.
2. Ouch! That soup is hot.
3. Oops! The plate broke.
4. Well, I guess I'll go.
5. Hurray! We won the game.
6. Wow! John hit the ball far.
7. Hurry! I saw something scary in the cave.
8. Alas! I cannot go with you.
9. Shh! I heard something.
10. Ah, I see what you mean.

Fill in the blanks with the correct INTERJECTIONS given below.

Eek!, Oh!, Oops!, Wow!, Hey!, Aha!, Ouch!, Ah!, Well, Ugh!

1. _____ He stole my watch.
2. _____ That hurts.
3. _____ I think I'll go.
4. _____ I hate rats.
5. _____ What a cute kitten.
6. _____ I lost my pencil.
7. _____ The bus left.
8. _____ How exciting.
9. _____ I guess you can have my soup.
10. _____ I slipped.

Answers				
1. Hey!	2. Ouch!	3. Well	4. Eek!	5. Aha!
6. Oh!	7. Ah!	8. Wow!	9. Well!	10. Oops

DETERMINERS

We use a number of words before common nouns (or adjective common noun) which we call determiners because they affect (or 'determine') the meaning of the noun. Determiners make it clear for example which particular thing(s) we are referring to or how much of a substance we are talking about. Singular countable nouns must normally have a determiner before them.

Determiners which classify or identify

Indefinite article	I bought a new pen yesterday
Definite article	The book I am reading is expensive
Demonstratives	I bought this/that table yesterday
Possessives	do you like my new car?

Determiners which indicate quantity

Numbers	I bought two new dresses yesterday.
Quantifiers	I didn't buy many apples today.

There wasn't much sugar in the house.

Determiners compared with pronouns

Determiners are always followed by a noun, words such as some and this followed by a noun function as determiners. When they stand on their own they function as pronouns:

I want some water (some+noun, functioning as determiner)

I want this   I want some

Important Determiners

Articles: a, an, the

Demonstratives: this, these, that, those

Possessives: my, our, your, his, her, its, their

Some other determiners: some, any, much, many, many a, each every, few, a few, the few, little, the little, a little either, neither, all, whole, less, fewer

Some, any

Some, when used with nouns to represent things that can be counted means a few or a small number. When used with a singular noun to represent something that cannot be counted 'some' means a little or a small quantity. Some is generally used in affirmative sentences as:

- ✓ I have bought some shirts.
- ✓ Some men are born great.

Any expresses a small number with countable nouns and a small quantity with singular uncountable nouns. Any is used in this sense in questions and negative sentences:

- ✓ Are there any files on my table?
- ✓ Is there any tea in the kettle?

Much, many

Many mean a great number. Much means a large quantity. Many is used with countable nouns. Much is used with uncountable nouns; as,

- ✓ Many people went to see the film.
- ✓ I do not have many books.

Less, fewer

Less denotes quantity; as,

- ✓ Please put less sugar in my coffee.
- ✓ He had less money in his pocket.

Fewer denotes number; as,

- ✓ There are fewer boys in this section than in that section.
- ✓ No fewer than twenty girls were absent today.

All, whole

All denotes number as well as quantity; as,

- ✓ He ate up all the sweets.
- ✓ All men are mortal.

Whole and the whole denote quantity only; as

- ✓ We have written the whole page.
- ✓ The whole of the shop is on fire.

Each, every

Each refers to one of two or more things or persons, the emphasis being on the individual whole of a group of more than two taken individually.

- ✓ Each girl will get a prize.
- ✓ Each student was given a book.

Either, neither

Either means one of the two or both, as,

- ✓ There are trees, on either side of the road.
- ✓ You can go by either road.

Neither means not either or none of the two; as,

- ✓ Neither side is winning.
- ✓ She took neither side.

Few, a few, the few

'Few' means hardly any. It has a negative meaning:

- ✓ Few men reach the age of a hundred years.
- ✓ Few people are free from faults.

A few means a small number. It has a positive meaning:

- ✓ He was asked to say a few words.
- ✓ The few means not many, but all of them.
- ✓ He lost the few friends he had.
- ✓ The few clothes the tailor had were spoilt.

Little, a little, the little

- ✓ Little means hardly any.

There is little hope of the patient's recovery.

- ✓ There is little sugar left in the pot.
- ✓ A little means some, though not much.
- ✓ He has still a little money left in the bank.
- ✓ A little knowledge is a dangerous thing.
- ✓ The little means not much, but the whole of it:
- ✓ I gave to the beggar the little money I had.

EXERCISE

Fill in the blanks with some, any, each, every, either and neither in the following:

- ❏ _____ side has won.
- ❏ _____ day has its problems.
- ❏ It rained _____ day during the holidays.
- ❏ We have_____ money.
- ❏ We do not have _____ rice.
- ❏ You may have _____ of the three books.
- ❏ _____ players did his best.
- ❏ He may take_____ side.
- ❏ Will you bring me _____ honey?
- ❏ _____ man must do his duty.

Fill in the blanks with many, much, all, whole and the whole in the following:

- ❏ _____ students attended the class.
- ❏ She had _____ wealth.
- ❏ The boxer ate the _____ loaf.
- ❏ _____ are not lovers of nature.
- ❏ We received _____help from our neighbours.
- ❏ The _____ family was plunged in grief.
- ❏ _____ men are mortal.
- ❏ _____ a boy was present today.
- ❏ Tagore has written ___ books.
- ❏ I ate a _____ pineapple.

TENSES AND THEIR USES

We all know that grammar is an essential part of English communication and conversation. Without Grammar, one cannot read or write the English language correctly.

Tenses are one of the most important aspects of reading and writing correct English language.

In Grammar, a tense is basically the time of a verb's action or state of being, such as present, past, or future. In other words, the verb of a tense shows the time of the action or work done, or being done. Primarily, there are **three tenses** – such as **The Present, Past and Future.** Look at the following sentences:

1. I <u>go</u> to school daily. (Present Tense)
2. I <u>went</u> to school yesterday. (Past Tense)
3. I <u>will</u> go to school tomorrow. (Future Tense)

Present Simple (I do.)

❑ We use this tense to talk about things in general:
  ✓ Doctors <u>treat</u> patients in hospitals. (Plural subject)
  ✓ The sun <u>rises</u> in the east. (Singular subject)
❑ To show habitual action:
  ✓ She <u>goes</u> to office daily at 10 o' clock.
  ✓ He <u>drinks</u> tea three times a day.
❑ To show a fixed action in future:
  ✓ The bus <u>leaves</u> at 4.30 in the morning.
  ✓ This TV serial <u>starts</u> at 8 p.m.

> **Note**
>
> *Only the first form of the verb is used in these sentences. Also, some verbs use 's' or 'es' after them according to the subject. In this case, helping verbs like 'is' or 'am' are not used with them. For example: I go (correct). I am not go (wrong).*

❑ To make negative and interrogative sentences, we use <u>do</u> and <u>does</u>:
  ✓ The bus <u>does not /doesn't</u> leave at 4.30.
  ✓ <u>Does</u> the bus leave at 4.30?

- ✓ Doctors <u>do not /don't</u> treat patents in hospitals.
- ✓ <u>Do</u> you eat meat?
- ✓ No, I <u>do not/ don't</u> eat meat.

Present Continuous (I am doing.)

❏ We use this tense to show an action going on but not finished:
- ✓ The boys <u>are playing</u> cricket in the field.
- ✓ I <u>am reading</u> a novel.

❏ We also use this tense to show an action about to happen in the near future:
- ✓ We <u>are eating</u> out tonight.
- ✓ My father <u>is coming</u> home early today.

> **Note**
>
> *Plural subjects are followed by <u>are,</u> while singular ones are followed by <u>is</u>. <u>I</u> takes <u>am</u> after it. In interrogative sentences, these verbs are put at the beginning. <u>Not</u> is placed after <u>is</u>, <u>am</u>, or <u>are</u>.*

- ✓ Are we <u>going</u> out tonight?
- ✓ No, we <u>are not/aren't</u>.

Present Perfect (I have done.)

❏ It shows or reflects completed activities connected with the present time or tense:
- ✓ I <u>have lost</u> my purse.
- ✓ He <u>has finished</u> his homework.

❏ It also denotes an action that had begun in the past and is having connection with the present:
- ✓ They <u>have lived</u> in this house <u>for</u> ten years.
- ✓ I <u>have known</u> this person <u>for</u> a long time.
- ✓ He <u>has been</u> absent <u>since</u> the last week.
- ✓ There <u>has been</u> an accident and the police are all around.
- ✓ I am dressing, I <u>haven't left</u> home yet.

> **Note**
>
> *Has, have, along with, been or the third form of verb are used. <u>Since</u> is used before definite time and <u>for</u> is used for a tentative period of time.*

Present Perfect Continuous (I have been doing.)

❏ This tense is generally used to express on activity which was continuing but has recently stopped:
- ✓ I <u>have been working</u> on this project <u>since</u> long but it seems to have reached a dead end.

- It also shows actions repeated over a period of time:
  - ✓ He <u>has</u> <u>been</u> playing cricket <u>since</u> he was ten.
- It expresses activities which began at some time and are still continuing:
  - ✓ He <u>has</u> <u>been</u> <u>working</u> at internet <u>for</u> six hours. (and is still continuing)

Note *This tense takes on or adopts 'has been/ have been' according to the subject followed by the verb, 'ing'.*

Past Simple (I did.)
- It denotes an action completed in past:
  - ✓ I <u>left</u> this house last year.
- It also denotes a past habit:
  - ✓ He always <u>shouted</u> at people.

Note *This tense is formed by using second 'for' in of verb.*

- <u>Did</u> *is used in interrogative and negative sentences:*
  - ✓ <u>Did</u> you go to office yesterday?
  - ✓ No, I didn't.

Note *With <u>did</u>, only the first form of the verb is used, 'did' is not used with <u>was/were</u>.*

Past Continuous (I was doing.)
- It denotes an action going on at a certain time which has not yet finished:
  - ✓ We <u>were</u> <u>watching</u> TV shows all night.
- To show some persistent past habit:
  - ✓ He <u>was</u> always <u>complaining</u>.
- *Past simple and past continuous are often used together:*
  - ✓ I hurt myself when I was practising long jump.

Note <u>*Was/were*</u> *are used in this tense along with the verb, 'ing' to show continuous action.*

Past Perfect (I had done.)
- *This tense is used to denote an action completed in the past before a certain moment:*
  - ✓ When I woke up in the morning, my father had already left for office.

Past Perfect Continuous (I had been doing.)

❑   It denotes an action that began at some point in the past and continued up to that time:

    ✓   I felt very irritated when I reached home, I <u>had</u> <u>been</u> travelling nearly for 12 hours.

<u>Had</u> <u>been</u> and <u>verb+ing</u> are used in this tense. The first action is in the past perfect continuous tense, while the second action is in simple past tense. Rules for since/ for are same as mentioned earlier.

Future Simple (I will do.)

❑   It expresses some future act:

    ✓   We <u>will</u> <u>win</u> the match.

    ✓   She <u>will</u> <u>go</u> to school tomorrow.

❑   *It is also used for offering or promising to do something*:

    ✓   I <u>will</u>/ <u>I'll</u> <u>help</u> you with this sum.

    ✓   <u>I'll</u> sure <u>lend</u> you some money.

❑   *Instead of <u>will,</u> use <u>going to</u> when you have decided to do something:*

    ✓   **Q.1.** When <u>will</u> you go on vacation?

    ✓   **A.1** I <u>am</u> <u>going to</u> Shimla next week.

❑   Going to/About to is also used in actions which are about to happen:

    ✓   Get into the bus. It is <u>going to</u>/ <u>about to</u> leave.

❑   Simple present tense is used instead of future tense for timetables.

    ✓   The school opens on 1ˢᵗ of July.

❑   In the 'if' clauses, will is not repeated.

    ✓   I'll go if it stops raining (not: will stop)

'Shall' and 'will' are always used with the first form of the verb.

Future Continuous (I will be doing.)

❑   *This kind of tense is generally used to denote actions which will be in progress in future or for an action already planned:*

    ✓   <u>I'll</u> <u>be</u> <u>taking</u> exam by this time tomorrow.

✓ I'll be staying in Kerala till next week.

❑ *For a planned action:*
✓ I am going to London next week. (not: will go)

❑ For official programs, 'is to' is used:
✓ The prime minister is to arrive tomorrow.

Will be takes verb + ing after it, and is to is followed by the first form of verb.

Future Perfect (I will have done.)

❑ It is used to denote an action or work that will be completed sometime in future:
✓ I shall have reached Mumbai by this time tomorrow.

In this tense, shall have/will have along with the third form of the verb are used.

Future Perfect Continuous (I will have been doing.)

❑ It denotes continuing actions is future and also their end:
✓ I'll have been living in this house for ten years next April.

In this tense, will/ shall have been along with the verb + ing are used.

	Simple/ Indefinite	Continuous	Perfect	Perfect Continuous
Present	He goes to school. (Affirmative) He doesn't go to school. (Negative) Does he go to school? (Interrogative) Doesn't he go to School? (Negative Interrogative)	He is going to school. He isn't going to school. Is he going to school? Isn't he going to school?	He has gone to school. He has not/hasn't gone to school. Has he gone to school? Hasn't he gone to school?	He has been going to school for two years. He has not been going to school for two years. Has he been going to school for two years? Hasn't he been going to school for two years?

Past	He went to school. Did he go to school? No, he didn't go to school.	He was going to school. Was he going to school? No, he wasn't going to school.	He had gone to school. Had he gone to school? No, he hadn't gone to school.	He had been going to school for two years. Had he been going to school for two years? No, he hadn't been going.....
Future	He will go to school tomorrow. Will he go to school tomorrow? No, he will not/won't go to school tomorrow.	He will be going to school tomorrow. Will he be going to school tomorrow? No, he won't be going to school tomorrow.	He will have gone to school. Will he have gone to school? No, he won't have gone to school.	He will have been going to school for two years. Will he have been going to school for two years? No, he won't have been going.....

Note

'am going to do' (something) or 'is going to do' are used in place of 'will be going' when we have already decided to do something or we have arranged do it.

In questions shall is used with I/we and will is used with you.

EXERCISE

Fill in the blanks with the correct forms of the following verbs. Use Simple Present Tense in each case.

(go, kill, do, eat, buy, go, agree, know)

1. We _____ not _____ overripe and cheap fruit.
2. _____ you _____ me?
3. He _____ not _____ meat.
4. I _____ not _____ with him
5. We daily _____ to school.
6. Rash driving _____ many people every year.

Answers					
1. do, buy	2. do, know	3. does, eat	4. do agree	5. go	6. kills

Complete the sentences with the correct forms of the verbs given below. Use Present Continuous Tense in each case.

solve, grow, go, insult, sell

1. I _____ _____ a puzzle. (What are you doing?)
2. Fruits _____ _____ on the trees. (What is growing on trees?)
3. I _____ _____ on the market. (Where are you going?)
4. _____ you _____ me? (What are you doing?)
5. He _____ _____ rotten fruit (what kind of fruit is he selling?)

Answers				
1. am solving	2. are growing	3. am going	4. are insulting	5. is selling

Put the correct forms of verbs given below. Use the Present Perfect Tense in each case.

stop, see, finish, come, stop, arrive

1. _____ you _____ writing your article? No, I _____.
2. She _____ _____ weeping.
3. _____ you _____ my brother?
4. I _____ just _____ my lunch.

5.   _____ he _____ home?
6.   The bus _____ _____.

Put in the correct forms of the following verbs and fill in the blanks suitably. Use the Present Perfect Continuous Tense in each case.

read, sit, swim, play, sit

1.   How long _____ you _____ _____ this book?
2.   I _____ _____ _____ the book for two hours.
3.   Where have you been? _____ you _____ _____?
4.   I _____ _____ _____ cricket since 4 o' clock.
5.   He _____ _____ _____ here all day.

Put in the correct forms of the following verbs and fill in the blanks. Use Simple Past Tense in each case.

Spend, fall, go, do, see, did(n't) drive, has spend

1.   Where _____ you _____ last night?
2.   I _____ to see a movie but I _____ enjoy it.
3.   _____ you _____ him yesterday? No, I _____.
4.   Last night he _____ down the stairs.
5.   Yesterday, he _____ rashly and _____ an accident
6.   Did you _____ all the money I _____ you?

Put in the correct forms of the following verbs and fill in the blanks below. Use Past Continuous Tense in each case.

Walk, watch, have, shed, are, is

1.   When I last saw him, he _____ _____ down the road very fast.

2. The trees _____ _____ leaves.
3. I _____ _____ in the park when. I met an old friend of mine.
4. I _____ _____ dinner yesterday at 8.30.
5. The door bell rang when I _____ _____ TV.

Put in the correct forms of the following verbs and fill in the blanks. Use Past Perfect Tense in each case.

Reach, die, break, eat, be

1. The patient _____ _____ before the doctor _____.
2. He was fasting, he _____ _____ nothing for a couple of days.
3. He was afraid to drive. He _____ never test _____ before.
4. When he _____ home, the thieves _____ _____ into the house.
5. It was my first visit to UK. I _____ never _____ there before.

Put in the correct forms of the following verbs and fill in the blanks. Use Past Perfect Continuous Tense in each case.

come, has be, has be, has be, ring, has be, live since/ for

1. I was in a bad mood when I _____ home. I _____ _____ working all day.
2. She cried in her sleep. She _____ _____ dreaming.
3. We _____ _____ taking the test for two hours when the bell _____.
4. The maid _____ _____ working in the house _____ two hours.
5. I _____ _____ _____ in this house since 2008.

Put in the correct forms of the following verbs and fill in the blanks. Use Simple Future Tense in each case.

Will, go, leave, shall, is going, will leave

1. The luggage looks heavy, I _____ help you unload it.

2. It is raining heavily. I don't think I _____ out tonight.
3. What time are you leaving for your trip abroad? I _____ _____ today evening. I have booked a seat in the plane.
4. This place looks horrible, I _____ not _____ to work here.
5. _____ I shut the door? It is very cold.
6. _____ you please shut the window?
7. He _____ _____ to buy a new bike.
8. I have got late. I think I _____ take a taxi.
9. _____ I go with you. It is quite dark out there.

Put in the correct forms of the following verbs and fill in the blanks. Use the Future Continuous Tense in each case.

See, take, read, make

1. The director _____ _____ _____ an announcement soon.
2. If you ring me at 10 o' clock, I _____ _____ _____ my lunch.
3. Right now he _____ _____ _____ a book in the library.
4. _____ you _____ _____ a bus or taxi for going home?
5. At this time tomorrow, I _____ _____ _____ a movie.

Put in the correct forms of the following verbs. Use only the Future Perfect Tense in each case.

Go, finish, start, leave

1. He won't be at home now. He _____ _____ _____ for office.
2. In a short while, the movie _____ _____ _____. All _____ _____ _____ home.
3. The show _____ _____ _____ by the time we reach the cinema hall.
4. Tomorrow they have their marriage anniversary. They _____ _____ _____ married for ten years.
5. The teacher _____ _____ _____ the course by the end of the term.
6. Don't speak until he _____ _____ .

Put in the correct forms of the following verbs. Use the Future Perfect Continuous Tense in each case.

Go, write, play, study, travel

1. He _____ _____ _____ cricket for four hours.
2. I _____ _____ _____ in this college for three years.
3. We _____ _____ _____ in the train for the last four hours.
4. He ___ _____ ____ the article since midnight.
5. The match _____ ____ ____ on for two hours now.

VOICE CHANGE (ACTIVE AND PASSIVE VOICE)

A Transitive verb has two voices: The **Active Voice** and the **Passive Voice**. The voice of a verb shows whether the subject is the receiver of the action (passive).

Compare the following sentences: Manish helped Ravi (active)/ Ravi was helped by Manish (passive). Both sentences mean the same thing, but in the first sentence Manish (the subject) is the doer of the action (helped) and in the second sentence, Ravi (the subject) is the receiver or sufferer of the action (was helped).

Use of Passive Voice

Though the active voice is more forceful and direct, the passive voice is used in the following conditions:

When we do not want to mention the doer of the action, as:

✓ She was found cheating.

When we do not know who is the doer of the action, as:

✓ My pocket has been picked.

When we want to emphasize the recipient of the action, as:

✓ The king was cheered by the people. / The old man was found dead.

CHANGING THE VOICE OF A VERB

We can change a sentence from active voice to passive voice by making the following changes:

The object in the active voice is made the subject in the passive voice.

The subject in the active voice is made the object in the passive voice.

The passive form of the verb is made by adding its past participle to some form of 'be' as shown in the following points:

SIMPLE PRESENT TENSE

He feeds pigeons. (Active)

Pigeons are fed by him. (Passive)

She teaches history. (Active)

History is taught by her. (Passive)

SIMPLE PAST TENSE

A snake bit Uma.

Uma was bitten by a snake.

I wrote a poem.

A poem was written by me.

SIMPLE FUTURE TENSE

Sasha will like this dress.

This dress will be liked by Sasha.

I shall cook dinner.

Dinner will be cooked by me.

CONTINUOUS TENSE (Present and Past)

They are watching a movie.

A movie is being watched by them.

A mad dog was chasing Mona.

Mona was being chased by a mad dog.

PERFECT TENSE (Present, Past and Future)

He has eaten a cake.

A cake has been eaten by him.

The hunter had killed a lion.

A lion had been killed by the hunter.

The teacher will have forgiven us.

We will have been forgiven by the teacher.

TRANSITIVE VERBS HAVING TWO OBJECTS

When a transitive verb has two objects in the active voice, either the direct or the indirect object may become the subject in the passive voice; as,

I gave Latika a pen.

Latika was given a pen by me.

A pen was given to Latika by me.

She will tell us a story.

We shall be told a story by her.

A story will be told to us by her.

PREPOSITIONAL VERBS

When the verb in the active voice is a prepositional verb, the preposition is not dropped in the passive voice, as it is a part of the verb; as,

The boys laughed at the beggar.

The beggar was laughed at by the boys.

We objected to the monitor's proposal.

The monitor's proposal was objected to by us.

AUXILIARY VERBS

You must do the job.

The job must be done by you.

Our team may lose the cricket match.

The cricket match may be lost by our team.

INTERROGATIVE SENTENCES

Has she taken a decision?

Has a decision been taken by her?

Who stole my watch?

By whom was my watch stolen?

IMPERATIVE SENTENCES

Shut the door.

Let the door be shut.

The door should be shut.

Let me complete my homework.

Let my homework be completed by me.

DOER OF THE ACTION

My wallet has been stolen.

Someone has stolen my wallet.

I was obliged to leave.

Circumstances obliged me to leave.

EXERCISE

Rewrite the following sentences according to the instructions given after each:

- ❏ The police caught the thief. (End: .... By the police)
- ❏ Too much is being taken for granted. (Begin: They are....)
- ❏ Who has broken the mirror? (Begin: By whom....)
- ❏ They must do it at once. (End:... done at once.)
- ❏ Someone has picked his pocket. (Begin: His pocket....)
- ❏ Passengers are forbidden to cross the line. (End:.... Forbids passengers to cross the line)
- ❏ Post this letter. (Begin: Let....)
- ❏ They feel that these situations need never arise. (End:.... felt that these situations need never arise).
- ❏ Will they help you? (End.... By them?)

Without adding 'by'; change the following sentences into Passive Voice:

- ❏ Somebody built this orphanage last year.
- ❏ People speak Hindi all over the world.
- ❏ No one has ever achieved greatness without sincere efforts.
- ❏ We called her stupid.
- ❏ Someone has stolen his water heater.
- ❏ People speak Assamese in Assam.
- ❏ They don't like newcomers in this village.
- ❏ They are serving cold drinks in the party.
- ❏ They drank a whole jug of juice.
- ❏ People always admire the brave.

Change the voice of the following sentences:

- ❏ Open the window.
- ❏ Her attitude shocked me a lot.
- ❏ The farmers are ploughing their fields.
- ❏ He landed the helicopter safely.
- ❏ My mother was feeding the birds.
- ❏ We are expecting rain.
- ❏ You should follow the advice of saints.

- [ ] Don't throw stones at the frogs.
- [ ] Take care of your health.

Change the following sentences into Active Voice. Frame at least two sentences following the pattern of each sentence given below.

- [ ] Hindi is spoken in India.
- [ ] The letter was given to me.
- [ ] You are requested not to cry.
- [ ] The poor should be fed.
- [ ] The children must be loved.
- [ ] The goods are carried by trucks.
- [ ] Nothing is to be gained.
- [ ] Kites were being flown.
- [ ] He was refused admission.
- [ ] They are being shown how to do it.
- [ ] This matter must be looked into.
- [ ] It is believed that the earth is round.
- [ ] I hope to be rewarded.
- [ ] She was paid her wages.
- [ ] I was helped.

NARRATION (DIRECT AND INDIRECT SPEECH)

There are two ways of relating what a person has said. We may quote his actual words. This is called direct speech. We may report what he said without quoting his exact words. This is called indirect speech.

- ✓ He said, "I am busy now." (Direct)
- ✓ He said that he was busy then. (Indirect)

Direct Speech
The actual words of a speaker are put within inverted commas. (" ")

The first word of a reported speech begins with a capital letter.

The reported speech is separated by a comma from the reporting verb.

Indirect Speech
Inverted commas are not used, but the conjunction 'that' is used

The comma separating the reporting verb from the reported speech is removed.

The tense of the reporting verb is never changed.

The question mark and the exclamatory mare are not used.

Interrogative imperative and exclamatory sentences are put as statements.

Assertive Sentences
Assertive sentences in the indirect speech are usually introduced by the conjunction 'that':

- ✓ They said to Anuj, "you are a brave boy."
- ✓ They told Anuj that he was a brave boy.

The verbs tell, inform, remind and assure always take a personal object after them, hence the form said to me is changed generally into told me and sometimes into informed me, reminded me, or assured me, as the sense may require; as,

The teacher said to me," I have never seen such a lazy girl as you are."

The teacher told me that she had never seen such a lazy girl as I was.

Imperative Sentences
When the direct speech is an imperative mood, the reporting verb say or tell is changed to some verb expressing a command, advice or request.

The imperative mood is changed into the infinitive.

The rules for the change of pronouns are to be observed.

That is generally not used. If it is used, then should is placed before the imperative instead of 'to'

When let in the direct speech expresses a proposal or suggestion, you may use should and change the reporting verb into propose or suggest; as,

- ✓ Direct: He said to us, "let us have some coffee."
- ✓ Indirect: He proposed to us that we should have some coffee.
- ✓ Direct: The teacher said to the pupils, "Do not stand here."
- ✓ Indirect: the teacher forbade the students to stand there.

Exclamatory Sentences

In reporting a wish or an exclamation in the indirect speech:

The reporting verb say or tell is changed into wish bless, pray, cry, exclaim, declare, confess, cry out etc., with such phrases as with regret with delight or joy with sorrow where necessary.

- ✓ Direct: He said, "God save my son!"
- ✓ Indirect: He prayed that God might save his son.
- ✓ Direct: "What a horrible accident it is!" he said.
- ✓ Indirect: He exclaimed that it was a horrible accident.

Interrogative Sentences

In reporting a question in the indirect speech:

The reporting verb is changed to asked, inquired, demanded. Etc.

The note of interrogation which is placed after questions in the direct form is replaced by a full stop.

- ✓ Direct: He said to me, "Do you know the way?"
- ✓ Indirect: He inquired of me if I knew the way.

Rewrite the following in Direct Speech:

- ❑ The boy asked me how old I was.
- ❑ The stranger asked Ashish where he lived.
- ❑ Ramu asked Nitin whether he had made a mistake.
- ❑ They asked me what I wanted.
- ❑ The young mouse asked who would bell the cat.
- ❑ I asked Nihal if he would lend me a pen.
- ❑ The policeman inquired of the girl where she was going.
- ❑ She enquired of us whether we were playing football.

CHAPTER 15

MODALS OR MODAL AUXILIARY VERBS

It is rude to say to a stranger, "Open the door," Normally, you would say to him:

"*Will* you open the door" Or "*would* you open the door?" Or "*could* you open the door?"

Verbs such as *would, will* and *could* are called *Modal Auxiliary Verbs* or *Modals.* These are often used to produce a particular effect and the modal you choose depends on several factors, such as the relationship you have with your listener, the formality or informality of the situation, and the importance of what you are saying.

Here is a list of the modals used in English:

Can,	*could,*	*may,*	*might,*	*must,*	*ought to,*	
Shall,	*should,*	*will ,*	*would*	*Dare*	*need,*	*need to*

Dare, *need to* and *used to* are called **semi-modals**.

Characteristics of Modals

Modals are called defective verbs because they cannot be used in all tenses and moods.

Study the following sentences:

- He might come soon.
- You should learn your lessons.
- I can sing that song.
- She must do her work.

We notice from these sentences that

- A modal verb is never used alone. It must have a principal verb with as,
  - ✓ Might come, should learn
- The modal verb used in the present tense have the same form throughout, whatever be the person and the number of the subject as,
  - ✓ I can sing. You can sing. He/she can sing. They can sing.
  - ✓ I may read. You may read. He/she may read. They may read.
- The modals do not have the infinitive or participle forms. We do not say: to shall, to must, to may etc.
  - ✓ However, in cases where we write to will, to dare, to need, etc. the verbs will, dare and need are used as principal verbs and not as Modal Auxiliaries.

✓ Let's consider the use of modals one by one.

Shall

1. In Assertive sentences, *shall*, in the first person, gives information about the future action; as,
   - ❑ I *shall* be much obliged to you.
   - ❑ We *shall* reach Delhi today.
2. *Shall*, in the second and third persons, is used to denote:
   - ❑ A *promise*; as,
     - ✓ She *shall* have the book tomorrow
     - ✓ They *shall* have a holiday tomorrow.
   - ❑ A *command*; as
     - ✓ They *shall* not play there.
     - ✓ You *shall* love your neighbor as yourself.
   - ❑ *Determination*; as,
     - ✓ They *shall* work hard.
     - ✓ You *shall* do what he has told you.
   - ❑ A *threat*; as,
     - ✓ He *shall* be punished if he does not obey them.
     - ✓ They *shall* pay for this negligence.
3. In interrogative sentences *shall*, used in the first person, indicates simple futurity, wish or opinion of the person spoken to; as,
   - ❑ *Shall* I buy this book for you?
     (Do you wish that I should buy this book for you?)
   - ❑ *Shall* we visit the museum?
     (Do you permit us to visit the museum?)

Will

1. In Assertive Sentences, *will* in the second and the third persons, indicates pure future; as,
   - ❑ She *will* go to Kanpur on Monday.
   - ❑ They are confident you *will* pass the examination.
2. In Assertive sentences, *will* indicates a customary or characteristic action, when used in the second or the third person; as,
   - ❑ She *will* sit there for hours waiting for her son to come.
   - ❑ Whenever he is in trouble, he *will* go to his father.
3. *Will*, in the second and third persons, expresses a belief or an assumption on the part of the speaker; as,
   - ❑ They *will* know it.

❑   Mohit *will* be back now.

4.   *Will,* in the first person is used to denote

    ❑   Promise; as

         ✓   We *will* do better next time.

         ✓   I *will* teach him math.

    ❑   Threat; as,

         ✓   I *will* dismiss you.

         ✓   We *will* expose her.

    ❑   Willingness; as,

         ✓   Don't worry; we *will* lend you some money.

         ✓   I *will* carry your bag to office.

    ❑   Determination; as,

         ✓   I *will* succeed in the venture.

         ✓   We *will* not surrender.

    ❑   In Interrogative sentences, *will* in the second person, denotes willingness, intention or wish of the person spoken to; as,

         ✓   *Will* you have a cup of coffee?

         ✓   *Will* you leave Mumbai on Sunday?

Should

Should is used:

1.   To denote duty or obligation; as,

         ✓   We should obey our elders.

         ✓   She should control her temper.

2.   To denote a condition, supposition, possibility, etc; as,

         ✓   If it should rain, we shall have a holiday.

         ✓   If he should come, ask him to wait.

3.   To indicate a concession; as,

         ✓   We will not believe it though an angel should come from heaven and say it.

4.   When giving and asking advice; as,

         ✓   You should not play with fire.

         ✓   You should forgive those who hurt you.

5.   After 'lest' to express a negative purpose; as,

         ✓   He worked hard lest he should fail.

6.   To disapprove something that was done in the past; as,

         ✓   They should not have laughed at her.

✓ I should not have gone for the picnic.

7.   In Idiomatic expression; as,

      ✓ He should think so. (He is quite sure of it)

Would

Would is used:

- ☐   To express determination: as,
    - ✓ She would have her own way.
    - ✓ The doctor said he would visit my ailing father every day.
- ☐   To express a wish; as,
    - ✓ I would like to see his house.
- ☐   To express frequent past actions; as,
    - ✓ After lunch he would have a short nap.
    - ✓ He would sit for hours watching the stars.
- ☐   To indicate refusal; as,
    - ✓ The wound would not heal quickly.
    - ✓ The engine would not start.
- ☐   In polite expressions; as,
    - ✓ Would you mind explaining this to me?
    - ✓ Would you please lend me some money?
- ☐   To denote condition or uncertainty; as,
    - ✓ Had he met me I would have told him everything.
    - ✓ If he were clever, he would resist this offer.

May

May is used:

- ☐   To express permission; as,
    - ✓ You may use my pen for the day.
    - ✓ May I come in, sir?
- ☐   To express a purpose; as,
    - ✓ She flatters so that she may win favors.
    - ✓ We eat that we may live.
- ☐   To denote possibility; as,
    - ✓ It may snow tonight.
    - ✓ I may be elected president.
- ☐   To express a wish; as,

- ✓ May you have the best of luck!
- ✓ May her soul rest in peace!

Might

- ❑ Might is used to denote a possibility that is more doubtful than 'may'; as,
  - ✓ She might pass.
  - ✓ The patient might recover.
- ❑ Might is also used to denote extreme politeness during a discussion as: Might I have a chance to speak?
  - ✓ If I might request you, couldn't you teach us history?
- ❑ Might is used to denote a gentle reproach or admonition; as,
  - ✓ Well, if you were not well, you might have told me this before.
  - ✓ You might tell me the truth.

Can, could

- ❑ Can and could are used to express possibility, that is, some action or event is possible; as,
  - ✓ Can her statement be true?
  - ✓ We could succeed if we worked together.
- ❑ Can and could are used to express ability or power; as,
  - ✓ I can swim
  - ✓ She could dance well at the age of ten.
- ❑ Can and could are used to express permission; as,
  - ✓ Can I go to see a movie?
  - ✓ You can leave the office, now.
- ❑ Could sometimes do not indicate past time. It is also used to express a polite request; as,
  - ✓ Could I have your book?
  - ✓ Could I have a word with you?

Need

- ❑ As a principal verb, need is used in the sense of 'stand in need of' or 'require'; as,
  - ✓ She needs my help.
  - ✓ They do not need your help.
- ❑ As an auxiliary verb, it expresses necessity or obligation and is used only in the present tense (for all persons). It is used only in interrogative and negative sentences.

- ✓ In negative sentences:

  He need not seek my permission.

  We need not worry. We have been provided for.

- ✓ In interrogative sentences:

  Need she do it again?

  Need I go to the hospital today?

- ✓ © need as a modal auxiliary doesn't have a past form. The past is expressed with need have in questions and needn't have in negative sentences; as,

  Need they have gone on strike? (They did go on strike.)

  They needn't have bought this house.

Dare

Dare is used:

- ❑ To denote 'challenge' or 'defiance' in affirmative sentences; as,
  - ✓ How dare she behave in this manner?
  - ✓ He dares to call you a thief

- ❑ To denote 'venture' and courage' in negative sentences; as,
  - ✓ I dare not ask him to teach me.
  - ✓ She dares not tell him lies.

- ❑ To make interrogative sentences; as,
  - ✓ Dare he say such a thing to me?
  - ✓ Does he dare to imply that I am dishonest?

- ❑ Must
  - ✓ Must is used to express:

- ❑ Fixed determination; as,
  - ✓ I must have my money back.
  - ✓ She must learn physics.

- ❑ Necessity, compulsion or strong moral obligation; as,
  - ✓ We must be loyal to our country.
  - ✓ I must finish the work today.

- ❑ Inevitability; as,
  - ✓ One day man must die.

- ❑ Certainty or strong likelihood; as,
  - ✓ She must have died by this time
  - ✓ Mary must have missed the train.

- ❑ Duty; as,
  - ✓ We must pay our school fees on time.
  - ✓ A soldier must be loyal.
- ❑ Prohibition or command; as,
  - ✓ Students must not eat in the classroom.

Ought (to)

Ought (to) is used:

- ❑ To denote strong probability; as,
  - ✓ You ought to secure full marks in math.
- ❑ To denote duty; as,
  - ✓ We ought to love our country.
  - ✓ We ought not to walk on the lawn.

Used (to)

Used (to) is used:

- ❑ To express a discontinued habit; as,
  - ✓ She used to live in this house some years ago.
  - ✓ There used to be some trees in this field.
- ❑ To denote a repeated action; as,
  - ✓ When he was young he used to play football.
  - ✓ She used to dance before marriage.
- ❑ 'Used to' also means accustomed to: as,
  - ✓ I am not used to hard manual labor.
  - ✓ They are used to a cold climate.

EXERCISE

Fill in the blanks with 'shall', 'will', 'should' or 'would':
1. We _____ speak the truth.
2. A dog _____ always remains faithful to his master.
3. Amit said that he _____ not talk to her any more.
4. A self-respecting man_____ rather die than tell lies.
5. As you sow, so _____ you reap.
6. You _____ be punished if you don't do the work.
7. The old man is walking with care lest he _____ stumble.
8. If I were you, I _____ not do it.
9. If today is Saturday, tomorrow _____ be Sunday.

Fill in the blanks with 'need', 'used to', 'ought to', 'dare' or 'must'.
1. He _____ call on me today.
2. Pupil's _____respect their teachers.
3. How _____ you enter my house?
4. One _____ obey the traffic rules.
5. A judge ___- be honest.
6. He _____- to do this heavy work.
7. They ___-- go out on Sundays.
8. _____ I remind you of your promise?
9. It ___ be done with great care.
10. He _____ not write to his grandfather.

Fill in the blanks with 'must', 'needn't', 'can', 'could', 'may', 'might', 'ought to' and 'should':
1. _____ my friend live long!
2. You _____ have been more careful.
3. Criminals___ be punished.
4. She _____ speak French when she was seven years old.
5. It _____ happen, but I don't think it will.
6. A cook _____ prepare the food with care.
7. We _____ always obey our superiors.

8.   Visitors____ not go beyond this limit.

9.   I ____ help you if I have time.

10.   We ____ hear people talking in the hall.

Make as many sentences as you can with the words given in the table below and identify the modals by underlining them.

It is rude to say to a stranger, "Open the door," Normally, you would say to him:

   "*Will* you open the door" Or "*would* you open the door?" Or "*could* you open the door?"

   Verbs such as *would, will* and *could* are called *Modal Auxiliary Verbs* or *Modals*. These are often used to produce a particular effect and the modal you choose depends on several factors, such as the relationship you have with your listener, the formality or informality of the situation, and the importance of what you are saying.

Here is a list of the modals used in English:

Can,	*could,*	*may,*	*might,*	*must,*	*ought to,*	
Shall,	*should,*	*will ,*	*would*	*Dare*	*need,*	*need to*

Dare, *need to* and *used to* are called **semi-modals**.

Characteristics of Modals

Modals are called defective verbs because they cannot be used in all tenses and moods.

Study the following sentences:

He might come soon.

You should learn your lessons.

I can sing that song.

She must do her work.

We notice from these sentences that

❑   A modal verb is never used alone. It must have a principal verb with as,

   ✓   Might come, should learn

❑   The modal verb used in the present tense have the same form throughout, whatever be the person and the number of the subject as,

   ✓   I can sing. You can sing. He/she can sing. They can sing.

   ✓   I may read. You may read. He/she may read. They may read.

❑   The modals do not have the infinitive or participle forms. We do not say: to shall, to must, to may etc.

However, in cases where we write to will, to dare, to need, etc. the verbs will, dare and need are used as principal verbs and not as Modal Auxiliaries.

Let's consider the use of modals one by one.

Shall

- ❑ In Assertive sentences, *shall,* in the first person, gives information about the future action; as,
    - ✓ I *shall* be much obliged to you.
    - ✓ We *shall* reach Delhi today.
- ❑ *Shall*, in the second and third persons, is used to denote:
    - ✓ A *promise*; as,

        She *shall* have the book tomorrow

        They *shall* have a holiday tomorrow.
- ❑ A *command*; as
    - ✓ They *shall* not play there.
    - ✓ You *shall* love your neighbor as yourself.
- ❑ *Determination*; as,
    - ✓ They *shall* work hard.
    - ✓ You *shall* do what he has told you.
- ❑ A *threat*; as,
    - ✓ He *shall* be punished if he does not obey them.
    - ✓ They *shall* pay for this negligence.
- ❑ In interrogative sentences *shall*, used in the first person, indicates simple futurity, wish or opinion of the person spoken to; as,
    - ✓ *Shall* I buy this book for you?

        (Do you wish that I should buy this book for you?)
    - ✓ *Shall* we visit the museum?

        (Do you permit us to visit the museum?)

Will

- ❑ In Assertive Sentences, *will* in the second and the third persons, indicates pure future; as,
    - ✓ She *will* go to Kanpur on Monday.
    - ✓ They are confident you *will* pass the examination.
- ❑ In Assertive sentences, *will* indicates a customary or characteristic action, when used in the second or the third person; as,
    - ✓ She *will* sit there for hours waiting for her son to come.
    - ✓ Whenever he is in trouble, he *will* go to his father.
- ❑ *Will,* in the second and third persons, expresses a belief or an assumption on the part of the speaker; as,
    - ✓ They *will* know it.

✓ Mohit *will* be back now.

❑ *Will,* in the first person is used to denote
  ✓ Promise; as,
> We *will* do better next time.
>
> I *will* teach him math.

  ✓ Threat; as,
> I *will* dismiss you.
>
> We *will* expose her.

  ✓ Willingness; as,
> Don't worry; we *will* lend you some money.
>
> I *will* carry your bag to office.

  ✓ Determination; as,
> I *will* succeed in the venture.
>
> We *will* not surrender.

  ✓ In Interrogative sentences, *will* in the second person, denotes willingness, intention or wish of the person spoken to; as,
> *Will* you have a cup of coffee?
>
> *Will* you leave Mumbai on Sunday?

Should

Should is used:

❑ To denote duty or obligation; as,
  ✓ We should obey our elders.
  ✓ She should control her temper.

❑ To denote a condition, supposition, possibility, etc; as,
  ✓ If it should rain, we shall have a holiday.
  ✓ If he should come, ask him to wait.

❑ To indicate a concession; as,
  ✓ We will not believe it though an angel should come from heaven and say it.

❑ When giving and asking advice; as,
  ✓ You should not play with fire.
  ✓ You should forgive those who hurt you.

❑ After 'lest' to express a negative purpose; as,
  ✓ He worked hard lest he should fail.

❑ To disapprove something that was done in the past; as,

- ✓ They should not have laughed at her.
- ✓ I should not have gone for the picnic.
- ❑ In Idiomatic expression; as,
  - ✓ He should think so. (He is quite sure of it)

Would

Would is used:

- ❑ To express determination: as,
  - ✓ She would have her own way.
  - ✓ The doctor said he would visit my ailing father every day.
- ❑ To express a wish; as,
  - ✓ I would like to see his house.
- ❑ To express frequent past actions; as,
  - ✓ After lunch he would have a short nap.
  - ✓ He would sit for hours watching the stars.
- ❑ To indicate refusal; as,
  - ✓ The wound would not heal quickly.
  - ✓ The engine would not start.
- ❑ In polite expressions; as,
  - ✓ Would you mind explaining this to me?
  - ✓ Would you please lend me some money?
- ❑ To denote condition or uncertainty; as,
  - ✓ Had he met me I would have told him everything.
  - ✓ If he were clever, he would resist this offer.

May

May is used:

- ❑ To express permission; as,
  - ✓ You may use my pen for the day.
  - ✓ May I come in, sir?
- ❑ To express a purpose; as,
  - ✓ She flatters so that she may win favors.
  - ✓ We eat that we may live.
- ❑ To denote possibility; as,
  - ✓ It may snow tonight.
  - ✓ I may be elected president.

- ❏ To express a wish; as,
  - ✓ May you have the best of luck!
  - ✓ May her soul rest in peace!

Might

- ❏ Might is used to denote a possibility that is more doubtful than 'may'; as,
  - ✓ She might pass.
  - ✓ The patient might recover.
- ❏ Might is also used to denote extreme politeness during a discussion as: Might I have a chance to speak?
  - ✓ If I might request you, couldn't you teach us history?
- ❏ Might is used to denote a gentle reproach or admonition; as,
  - ✓ Well, if you were not well, you might have told me this before.
  - ✓ You might tell me the truth.

Can, could

- ❏ Can and could are used to express possibility, that is, some action or event is possible; as,
  - ✓ Can her statement be true?
  - ✓ We could succeed if we worked together.
- ❏ Can and could are used to express ability or power; as,
  - ✓ I can swim
  - ✓ She could dance well at the age of ten.
- ❏ Can and could are used to express permission; as,
  - ✓ Can I go to see a movie?
  - ✓ You can leave the office, now.
- ❏ Could sometimes do not indicate past time. It is also used to express a polite request; as,
  - ✓ Could I have your book?
  - ✓ Could I have a word with you?

Need

- ❏ As a principal verb, need is used in the sense of 'stand in need of' or 'require'; as,
  - ✓ She needs my help.
  - ✓ They do not need your help.
- ❏ As an auxiliary verb, it expresses necessity or obligation and is used only in the present tense (for all persons). It is used only in interrogative and negative sentences.
  - ✓ In negative sentences:

He need not seek my permission.

We need not worry. We have been provided for.

✓ In interrogative sentences:

Need she do it again?

Need I go to the hospital today?

❑ © need as a modal auxiliary doesn't have a past form. The past is expressed with need have in questions and needn't have in negative sentences; as,

✓ Need they have gone on strike? (They did go on strike.)

✓ They needn't have bought this house.

Dare

Dare is used:

❑ To denote 'challenge' or 'defiance' in affirmative sentences; as,

✓ How dare she behave in this manner?

✓ He dares to call you a thief

❑ To denote 'venture' and courage' in negative sentences; as,

✓ I dare not ask him to teach me.

✓ She dares not tell him lies.

❑ To make interrogative sentences; as,

✓ Dare he say such a thing to me?

✓ Does he dare to imply that I am dishonest?

Must

Must is used to express:

❑ Fixed determination; as,

✓ I must have my money back.

✓ She must learn physics.

❑ Necessity, compulsion or strong moral obligation; as,

✓ We must be loyal to our country.

✓ I must finish the work today.

❑ Inevitability; as,

✓ One day man must die.

❑ Certainty or strong likelihood; as,

✓ She must have died by this time

✓ Mary must have missed the train.

❑ Duty; as,

✓ We must pay our school fees on time.

- ✓ A soldier must be loyal.
- ❑ Prohibition or command; as,
  - ✓ Students must not eat in the classroom.

Ought (to)

Ought (to) is used:

- ❑ To denote strong probability; as,
  - ✓ You ought to secure full marks in math.
- ❑ To denote duty; as,
  - ✓ We ought to love our country.
  - ✓ We ought not to walk on the lawn.

Used (to)

Used (to) is used:

- ❑ To express a discontinued habit; as,
  - ✓ She used to live in this house some years ago.
  - ✓ There used to be some trees in this field.
- ❑ To denote a repeated action; as,
  - ✓ When he was young he used to play football.
  - ✓ She used to dance before marriage.
- ❑ 'Used to' also means accustomed to: as,
  - ✓ I am not used to hard manual labor.
  - ✓ They are used to a cold climate.

Fill in the blanks with 'shall, will, should or would':

- ❑ We _____ speak the truth.
- ❑ A dog _____ always remains faithful to his master.
- ❑ Amit said that he _____ not talk to her any more.
- ❑ A self-respecting man_____ rather die than tell lies.
- ❑ As you sow, so _____ you reap.
- ❑ You _____ be punished if you don't do the work.
- ❑ The old man is walking with care lest he _____ stumble.
- ❑ If I were you, I _____ not do it.
- ❑ If today is Saturday, tomorrow _____ be Sunday.

Fill in the blanks with 'need, used to, ought to, dare or must'.

❏ He _____ call on me today.

❏ Pupil's _____ respect their teachers.

❏ How _____ you enter my house?

❏ One _____ obey the traffic rules.

❏ A judge _____ be honest.

❏ He _____ to do this heavy work.

❏ They _____ go out on Sundays.

❏ _____ I remind you of your promise?

❏ It _____ be done with great care.

❏ He _____ not write to his grandfather.

Fill in the blanks with 'must', 'needn't', 'can', 'could', 'may', 'might', 'ought to' and 'should':

❏ _____ my friend live long!

❏ You _____ have been more careful.

❏ Criminals _____ be punished.

❏ She _____ speak French when she was seven years old.

❏ It _____ happen, but I don't think it will.

❏ A cook _____ prepare the food with care.

❏ We _____ always obey our superiors.

❏ Visitors _____ not go beyond this limit.

❏ I _____ help you if I have time.

❏ We _____ hear people talking in the hall.

THE GERUND

A gerund is a verbal noun which does the work of a verb and of a noun. A gerund being a verbal noun is used in the following ways:

- ❑ **As a subject of a verb, as:**
    - ✓ Cheating should be discouraged.
    - ✓ Smoking is bad for health.
- ❑ **As the object of a verb, as:**
    - ✓ She likes swimming.
    - ✓ All the boys started shouting.
- ❑ **As the object of a preposition, as:**
    - ✓ They were accused of stealing.
    - ✓ He was prevented from visiting the spot.
- ❑ **As the complement of a verb, as:**
    - ✓ What I dislike most is cheating.
    - ✓ My favourite pastime is bird watching.
- ❑ **Like a verb, it may take an object, as:**
    - ✓ She believes in talking trash.
    - ✓ We are fond of singing songs.

Gerund and Infinitive

Both the gerund and the infinitive are used in the same sense. They are formed form a verb and are used as nouns; as,

Sleeping is good for health (gerund)	To sleep is good for health. (Infinitive)
Seeing is believing (gerund)	To see is to believe.

Gerund and Present Participle

Both the Gerund and the Present Participle end in, –ing. The former is sued like a noun and the latter is sued like an adjective; as,

Sleeping is good for health (gerund)	A sleeping dog can be dangerous. (Present participle)
The old man was tired of walking. (Gerund).	Walking along the road, I met my friend. (Present Participle)

Put the verbs in brackets into the gerund form:

1. Sunita does not enjoy (go) to the dentist.
2. I hate (borrow) money.
3. Would you mind (write) your address on the form?
4. Stop (argue) and start (think).
5. He is thinking of (make) his will.
6. Is there anything there worth (buy)?
7. It's no use (cry) over spilt milk.
8. She is looking forward to (read) your article.
9. I remember (read) a review of that film.
10. He finished (speak) and left the hall.

Complete the sentences with the gerund form of the verbs in the parentheses given below. One has been done for you.

1. She is good at (dance).   .
2. He is crazy about (sing) .
3. I don't like (play) cards.
4. They are afraid of (swim) in the sea.
5. You should give up (smoke) .
6. Sam dreams of (be) a pop star.
7. He is interested in (make) friends.
8. My uncle is afraid of (go)   by plane.
9. We insist on (cook) the dinner ours

Locate the gerund in each sentence. Write your answer in the box below the sentence. Note: If the gerund is a part of a gerund phrase, include the whole phrase in your answer.

1. Hours of editing the newspaper ruined her day.

2. Hanging the pictures on the wall was more difficult than we had anticipated.

3. Try to slip away without telling your friends about it.

4. Each afternoon Miriam enjoyed swimming a few laps.

5. Winning at poker makes Don feel important.

6. I am demoting the officer for disobeying orders.

7. One of my favorite events is canoeing down the Mississippi River.

8. Sometimes wisdom simply means knowing about the importance of silence.

9. Without studying for the test, you are taking a big chance.

10. Abbey is enjoying listening to the Rolling Stones' music.

Answers

1. Editing the newspaper (gerund phrase) 2. Hanging the pictures on the wall

3. Telling your friends about it 4. Swimming a few laps

5. Winning at poker 6. Disobeying orders

7. Canoeing down the Mississippi River 8. Knowing about the importance of silence

9. Studying for the test 10. Listening to the Rolling Stones' music

DEGREES OF COMPARISON

An adjective of quality can be used in three degrees: positive, comparative and superlative. They are called the three degrees of comparison.

Positive:	This is a good book.
	Gold is a precious metal.
Comparative:	That book is better than your book.
	Gold is more precious than copper.
Superlative:	This book is the best of all books.
	Gold is the most precious of all metals.

Interchange of Degree of Comparison

1. Comparative: She is taller than I

   Positive   :   I am not as tall as she.

2. Superlative   :   Gaurav is the best boy in the class.

   Comparative   :   Gaurav is better than any other boy in the class.

   Positive   :   No other boy in the class is as good as Gaurav.

3. Superlative   :   Mumbai is the biggest town in India.

   Comparative: Mumbai is bigger than any other town in India.

Some Important Adjectives

❑ Elder, Older. Eldest, Oldest
  - ✓ He is my elder brother
  - ✓ His eldest son joined the army.
  - ✓ He is the oldest man in the village.

❑ Later, Latter, Latest, Last
  - ✓ He came later than I.
  - ✓ This is a later edition of the book.
  - ✓ This is the latest news.
  - ✓ Ravi and Harish are my friends. The former is a teacher, the latter is an artist.

- ✓ I could not hear the latter part of his speech.
- ✓ Ours is the last house in the street.

❑ *Farther, Further*
- ✓ Your house is farther from the school than mine.
- ✓ Chennai is farther from Delhi than Kolkata.

❑ *Nearest, Next*
- ✓ The thief was taken to the nearest police station.
- ✓ I am leaving by the next train.

❑ *Less, Fewer*
- ✓ I have less money than you.
- ✓ Mo fewer than sixty passengers were injured.
- ✓ No fewer than six attacks were made last night.

EXERCISE

Change the degree of comparison without changing the meaning:
1. Australia is the largest island in the world.
2. A wise enemy is better than a foolish friend.
3. Hunger is the best sauce.
4. Very few countries are as rich as America.
5. No other man is as strong as Atul.
6. Shakespeare is greater than any other English poet.
7. No other exercise is as convenient as swimming.
8. Hyderabad is not so cool as Bangalore.

Fill in the blanks with 'elder', 'eldest', 'older' or 'oldest':
1. He is the _____ man in our village.
2. She is my ___ sister.
3. He is the _____ of the two brothers.
4. She is _____ than Seema.
5. Rita is the ___ girls in the school.
6. This is the ___ temple in Goa.
7. She is _____ than my brother.
8. Of the two brothers Aseem is the _____.

TRANSFORMATION OF SENTENCES

Transformation is changing the form of a sentence without changing its meaning. In the exams, transformation should be done according to the direction given in the question paper. In doing transformation, a student should have a fairly good knowledge about the kinds of sentences and their formation. A brief direction about doing *transformation is given below.*

Affirmative to Negative:

Rule 1: Only/ alone/ merely → Replaced by → None but (person)/ nothing but(things)/ not more than or not less than(number)

❑ Eg.
- ✓ Affirmative: Only Allah can help us. Negative: None but Allah can help us.
- ✓ Affirmative: He has only a ball. Negative: He has nothing but a ball.
- ✓ Affirmative: He has only ten rupees. Negative: He has not more than ten rupees.

Rule 2: Must → Replaced by → Cannot but/ Cannot help+ (v+ing).

❑ Eg.
- ✓ Affirmative: We must obey our parents. Negative: We cannot but obey our parents/We cannot help obeying our parents.

Rule 3: Both----and → Replaced by → not only ---- but also.

❑ Ex:
- ✓ Aff: Both Dolon and Dola were excited.
- ✓ Neg: Not only dolon but also Dola were present.

Rule 4: and (if join two words) → Replaced by → Not only ----- but also.

❑ Ex:
- ✓ aff: He was obedient and gentle. Neg: He was not only obedient but also gentle.

Rule 5: Everyone/ everybody/every person/ (every + common noun)/all → Replaced by → There is no + attached word + but.

❑ Ex:
- ✓ Aff: Every mother loves her child.
- ✓ Neg: There is no mother but loves her child.

Rule 6: As soon as → Replaced by → No sooner had ----- Than.

- ❏ Ex:
  - ✓ Aff: As soon as the thief saw the police, he ran away. Neg: No sooner had the thief saw the police he ran away.

Rule 7: Absolute Superlative degree → Replaced by → No other+ attached word+so+ positive form+ as+subject.

- ❏ Ex:
  - ✓ aff: Dhaka is the biggest city in Bangladesh.
  - ✓ Neg: No other city is as big as Dhaka in Bangladesh.

Rule 8: Sometimes affirmative sentences are changed into negative by using opposite words. Before the word, off course 'not' is used.

- ❏ Ex:
  - ✓ Aff: I shall remember you. Neg: I shall not forget you.

Rule 9: Always → Replaced by → Never.

- ❏ Ex:
  - ✓ aff: Raven always attends the class. Neg: Raven never misses the class.

Rule 10: Too ---- to → Replaced by → so ---that+ can not/could not(in past).

- ❏ Ex:
  - ✓ Aff: He is too weak to walk. Neg: He is so weak that he cannot walk.

Rule 11: As – as → Replaced by → Not less – than.

- ❏ Ex:
  - ✓ Aff: Simi was as wise as Rimi. Neg: Simi was not less wise than Rimi.

Rule 12: Universal truth are change by making them negative interrogative.

- ❏ Ex:
  - ✓ Aff: The Sun sets in the west. Neg: Doesn't the Sun set in the west?

Rule 13: Sometimes → Replaced by → Not + always.

- ❏ Ex:
  - ✓ Aff: Raven sometimes visits me. Neg: Raven doesn't always visit me.

Rule 14: Many → Replaced by → Not a few.

- ❏ Ex:
  - ✓ Aff: I have many friends. Neg: I donot have few friends.

Rule 15: A few → Replaced by → not many.

- ❏ Ex:
  - ✓ Aff: Bangladesh has a few scholars. Neg: Bangladesh doesn't have many scholars.

Rule 16: Much → Replaced by → A little.

- ❑ Ex:
  - ✓ Aff: He belongs much money. Neg: He doesn't belong a little money.

Rule 17: A little → Replaced by → not much.

- ❑ Ex:
  - ✓ Aff: Dolon has a little riches. Neg: Dolon doesn't have much riches.

Assertive to Interrogative

Rule 1: If the sentence is in the affirmative, you have to change it into the negative interrogative. If it is in negative, then you have to change it into bare interrogative.

- ❑ Ex:
  - ✓ Ass: He was very gentle.
  - ✓ Int: Was n't he very gentle?
  - ✓ Aff: He is not a good person.
  - ✓ Int: Is he a good person?

Rule 2: No auxiliary verb in sentence →→ Change it by using →→ Do/does/did or Don't/doesn't/ didn't.

- ❑ Ex:
  - ✓ Ass:He plays Football.
  - ✓ Int: Does he play football?
  - ✓ Ass: They did not play football yesterday.
  - ✓ Int: Did they play football yesterday?

Rule 3: Never → Replaced by → Ever.

  - ✓ Ass: I never drink tea.
  - ✓ Int: Do I ever drink tea?

Rule 4: Everybody/everyone/ All → Replaced by → Who + Don't/ Doesn't/ Didn't

- ❑ Ex:
  - ✓ Everybody wishes to be happy.
  - ✓ Int : Who doesn't wish to be happy?

Rule 5: Every + noun → Replaced by → Is there any + noun+ Who don't/doesn't/didn't.

- ❑ Ex:
  - ✓ Ass: Every man wishes to be happy.
  - ✓ Int: Is there any man who doesn't wish to be happy?

Rule 6: No body/ no one / None → Replaced by → Who.

- ❑ Ex:
  - ✓ Nobody could count my love for you.

✓ Int: Who could ever count my love for you?

Rule 7: There is no → Replaced by → Is there any/ Who(person)/ What(thing).

   ❑   Ex:

        ✓ Ass: There is no use of this law.

        ✓ Int: What is the use of this law.

        ✓ Ass: There is no man happier than Jamil.

        ✓ Int: Who is Happier than jamil.

Rule 8: It Is no → Replaced by → Is there any/Why.

   ❑   Ex:

        ✓ Ass: It is no use of taking unfair means in the exam.

        ✓ Int: Why take unfair means in the exam? Or,

        ✓ Is there any use of this law?

Rule 9: It Doesn't matter → Replaced by → what though/ Does it matter.

   ❑   Ex:

        ✓ Ass: It does not matter if you fail in te exam.

        ✓ Int: What though if you fail in the exam?

        ✓ Interrogative to assertive is to be done doing vice versa.

Exclamatory to Assertive

Rule1: The Subject and Verb of the exclamatory sentence are to be used as the subject and the verb of the assertive sentence at the outset of the sentence.

How/What → Replace by → Very(before adjective)/ Great(before noun)

   ❑   Ex:

        ✓ How fortunate you are!

        ✓ Ass: You are very fortunate.

        ✓ Exc: What a fool you are!

        ✓ Ass: You are a great fool.

Rule 2: Sometimes the subject and verb may be eclipsed.

   ❑   Ex:

        ✓ What a beautiful scenery!

        ✓ Ass: It is a very beautiful scenery.

   ❑   Ex:

        ✓ What a pity!

        ✓ Ass: It is a great pity.

Rule 3: Hurrah/ Bravo → Replace by → I/we rejoice that/ It is a matter of joy that.

   ❑   Ex:

        ✓ Hurrah! We have own the game.

✓ Ass: It is a matter of joy that we have won the game.

Rule 4: Alas → Replace by → I/we Mourn that/ It is a matter of sorrow or grief that.

❑ Ex:

✓ Alas! He has failed.

✓ Ass: We mourn that he has failed.

Rule 5: Had/were/If /Would that (at the outset) → Replaced by → I wish + subject again + were/ had+ rest part.

❑ Ex:

✓ Had I the wings of a bird!

✓ Ass: I wish I had the wings of a bird.

❑ Ex:

✓ Were I a bird!

✓ Ass: I wish I were a bird.

❑ Ex:

✓ If I were young again!

✓ Ass: I wish I were young again.

❑ Ex:

✓ would that I could be a child!

✓ Ass: I wish I could be a child.

Assertive to Exclamatory is to be done doing the vice versa of the above.

Imperative to Assertive

Rule 1: Add subject + should in doing assertive.

❑ Ex:

✓ Do the work.

✓ Ass: you should do the work.

Rule 2: Please/kindly → Replaced by →You are requested to.

❑ Ex:

✓ Please, help me.

✓ Ass: You are requested to help me.

Rule 3: Do not → Replaced by → You should not.

❑ Ex:

✓ Do not run in the sun.

✓ Ass: you should not run in the sun.

Rule 4: Never → Replaced by → you should never.

❑ Ex:

✓ Never tell a lie.

    ✓ Ass: You should never tell a lie.

Rule 5: Let us → Replaced by → We should.

  ❑   Ex:

    ✓ Let us go out for a walk.

    ✓ Ass: We should go out for a walk.

Rule 6: Let + noun/pronoun → Replaced by → Subject + might.

  ❑   Ex:

    ✓ Let him play football.

    ✓ Ass: He might play football.

Sentences having the Adverb, 'Too'

    ✓ The dog is too old to learn new things.

    ✓ The dog is so old that it cannot learn new things.

    ✓ He is too clever not to see through your tricks.

    ✓ He is so clever that he sees through your tricks.

Interchanging of Degrees of Comparison

    ✓ He runs as fast as a deer. (Positive)

    ✓ A deer does not run faster than he. (Comparative)

    ✓ Hydrogen is the lightest of all gases. (Superlative)

    ✓ Hydrogen is lighter than any other gas. (Comparative)

    ✓ No gas is as light as hydrogen. (Positive)

Interchange of Active and Passive Voice

    ✓ I wrote a poem. (Active)

    ✓ A poem was written by me. (Passive)

    ✓ Who taught you French? (Active)

    ✓ By whom was French taught to you? (Passive)

Interchange of Parts of Speech

    ✓ *Noun:* The patient put up a brave fight.

    ✓ *Verb:* The patient fought bravely.

    ✓ *Noun:* It was her intention to tease me.

    ✓ *Adverb*: She teased me intentionally.

Interchange of Principal and Subordinate Clauses

    ✓ He is so weak that he cannot walk.

    ✓ He cannot walk as he is very weak.

    ✓ It never rains but pours.

✓ It always pours when it rains.

1. **Conversion of Simple Sentences into Compound Sentences**
   - ❏ Simple: The weather being fine, we went out for a walk.
   - ❏ Compound: The weather was fine and we went out for a walk.
   - ❏ Simple: Notwithstanding her old age, my mother works hard.
   - ❏ Compound: My mother is old but she works hard.

2. **Conversion of Compound Sentences into Simple Sentences**
   - ❏ Compound: He is poor, but he is happy.
   - ❏ Simple: In spite of his poverty, he is happy.
   - ❏ Simple: You must work hard to pass the examination.
   - ❏ Compound: The sun rose and the fog dispersed.
   - ❏ Simple: The sun having risen, the fog dispersed.

3. **Conversion of Compound Sentences into Complex Sentences**
   - ❏ Compound: Run fast, or you will miss the train.
   - ❏ Complex: Unless you run fast, you will miss the train.
   - ❏ Compound: He will come today and I have no doubt about it.
   - ❏ Complex: I have no doubt that he will come today.

4. **Conversion of Complex Sentences into Compound Sentences**
   - ❏ Complex: I have found the ring that I have lost.
   - ❏ Compound: I have lost her ring, but I have found it.
   - ❏ Complex: If you do not hurry you will miss the train.
   - ❏ Compound: You must hurry, or you will miss the train.

5. **Conversion of Simple Sentences into Complex Sentences**
   - ❏ *Noun Clauses*
     - ✓ Simple: No one can foretell the time of his death.
     - ✓ Complex: No one can foretell when he will die.
     - ✓ Simple: Her ambition was to become a doctor.
     - ✓ Complex: Her ambition was that she should become a doctor.
   - ❏ *Adjective Clauses*
     - ✓ Simple: All glittering things are not gold.
     - ✓ Complex: All that glitters is not gold.
     - ✓ Simple: A man in danger needs help.
     - ✓ Complex: A man who is in danger needs help.
   - ❏ *Adverb Clauses*
     - ✓ Simple: We eat to live.

- ✓ Complex: We eat so that we may live.
- ✓ Simple: I will go with your permission.
- ✓ Complex: I will go if you give me permission.

EXERCISE

Interchange the principal and the subordinate clauses in the following sentences:

- ❑ Look before you leap.
- ❑ As soon as the storm began, the boat capsized.
- ❑ Unless you work hard, you will not come up in life.
- ❑ He never makes a promise which he cannot keep.
- ❑ He ran away as soon as he saw me.
- ❑ I cannot speak loudly because I have a sore throat.
- ❑ I was so foolish that I did not act upon my teacher's advice.
- ❑ She does not like him because he is proud.
- ❑ No sooner did the bell ring than the boys ran into their classes.
- ❑ The money was not returned until the thief was beaten.

CHAPTER 19

IDIOMS AND IDIOMATIC EXPRESSIONS

What are Idioms?

Idioms are *words, phrases or expressions* which are commonly used in everyday conversation by native speakers of English. They are often *metaphorical* and make the language more *colourful*.

Example:- Let the cat out of the bag: If you let the cat out of the bag, means you reveal a secret.

It is important to remember that idiomatic expressions are used when speaking informally. They are **not** used in formal exchanges.

List of Some Commonly Used Idioms

Add fuel to the flames:	If you *add fuel to the flames*, you do or say something that makes a difficult situation even worse. He forgot their wedding anniversary, and his apologies only added fuel to the flames.
All ears:	To say that you are *all ears* means that ou are listening very attentively. Of course, I want to know - I'm all ears!
Answer the call of nature or the nature's call:	When a person *answers the call of nature*, they go to the toilet. I had to get up in the middle of the night to answer the call of nature.
Backseat driver:	A passenger in a car who gives unwanted advice to the driver is called a *backseat driver.* *I can't stand backseat drivers like my mother-in-law!*
Badger someone:	If you *badger someone* into doing something, you persistently nag or pester them until you obtain what you want. Sophie badgered her parents into buying her a new computer.
Balancing act:	When you try to satisfy two or more people or groups who have different needs, and keep everyone happy, you perform a *balancing act*. Many people, especially women, have to perform a balancing act between work and family.

Bare your heart/soul:	If you *bare you soul* (or heart) to someone, you reveal your inner-most thoughts and feelings to them. Mike couldn't keep things to himself any longer. He decided to bare his soul to his best friend.
Bark up the wrong tree	A person who is *barking up the wrong tree* is doing the wrong thing, because their beliefs or ideas are incorrect or mistaken. The police are barking up the wrong tree if they think Joey stole the car - he can't drive!
Beat a (hasty) retreat:	Someone who *beats a (hasty) retreat* runs away or goes back hurriedly to avoid a dangerous or difficult situation. The thief beat a hasty retreat as soon as he saw the security officer.
One's best bet:	The action most likely to succeed is called one's *best bet.* *Your best bet would be to try calling him at home.*
Bide your time:	If you *bide your time*, you wait for a good opportunity to do something. He's not hesitating, he's just biding his time, waiting for the price to drop.
Binge drinking:	This term refers to heavy drinking where large quantities of alcohol are consumed in a short space of time, often among young people in rowdy groups. Binge drinking is becoming a major problem in some European countries.

Bird In The Hand Is Worth Two In The Bush:

❑ Having something that is certain is much better than taking a risk for more, because chances are that you might lose everything.

❑ A Blessing In Disguise: Something good that isn't recognized at first.

A Chip On Your Shoulder:

❑ Being upset for something that happened in the past.

A Dime A Dozen:

❑ Anything that is common and easy to get.

A Doubting Thomas:

❑ A skeptic who needs physical or personal evidence in order to believe something.

A Drop in the Bucket:

❑ A very small part of something big or whole.

A Fool And His Money Are Easily Parted:

❑ It's easy for a foolish person to lose his/her money.

A House Divided Against Itself Cannot Stand:
- ❑ Everyone involved must unify and function together or it will not work out.

A Leopard Can't Change His Spots:
- ❑ You cannot change who you are.

A Penny Saved Is A Penny Earned:
- ❑ By not spending money, you are saving money (little by little).

A Picture Paints a Thousand Words:
- ❑ A visual presentation is far more descriptive than words.

A Piece of Cake:
- ❑ A task that can be accomplished very easily.

A Slap on the Wrist:
- ❑ A very mild punishment.

A Taste Of Your Own Medicine:
- ❑ When you are mistreated the same way you mistreat others.

A Toss-Up:
- ❑ A result that is still unclear and can go either way.

Actions Speak Louder Than Words:
- ❑ It's better to actually do something than just talk about it.

Add Fuel To The Fire:
- ❑ Whenever something is done to make a bad situation even worse than it is.

Against The Clock:
- ❑ Rushed and short on time.

All Bark And No Bite:
- ❑ When someone is threatening and/or aggressive but not willing to engage in a fight.

All Greek to me:
- ❑ Meaningless and incomprehensible like someone who cannot read, speak, or understand any of the Greek language would be.

All In The Same Boat:
- ❑ When everyone is facing the same challenges.

An Arm And A Leg:

❑　　Very expensive. A large amount of money.

An Axe To Grind:

❑　　To have a dispute with someone.

Apple of My Eye:

❑　　Someone who is cherished above all others.

As High As A Kite:

❑　　Anything that is high up in the sky.

At The Drop of A Hat:

❑　　Willing to do something immediately.

Back to Square One:

❑　　Having to start all over again.

Back To The Drawing Board:

❑　　When an attempt fails and it's time to start all over.

Baker's Dozen:

❑　　Thirteen.

Beat A Dead Horse:

❑　　To force an issue that has already ended.

Beating Around The Bush:

❑　　Avoiding the main topic. Not speaking directly about the issue.

Bend Over Backwards:

❑　　Do whatever it takes to help. Willing to do anything.

Between A Rock And A Hard Place:

❑　　Stuck between two very bad options.

Bite Off More Than You Can Chew:

❑　　To take on a task that is way to big.

Bite Your Tongue:

❑　　To avoid talking.

Blood Is Thicker Than Water:

❑　　The family bond is closer than anything else.

Blue Moon:

❑　　A rare event or occurance.

Break A Leg:

❑　　A superstitious way to say 'good luck' without saying 'good luck', but rather the opposite.

Buy A Lemon:
- ❏ To purchase a vehicle that constantly gives problems or stops running after you drive it away.

Can't Cut The Mustard:
- ❏ Someone who isn't adequate enough to compete or participate.

Cast Iron Stomach:
- ❏ Someone who has no problems, complications or ill effects with eating anything or drinking anything.

Charley Horse:
- ❏ Stiffness in the leg/A leg cramp.

Chew Someone Out:
- ❏ Verbally scold someone.

Chip on his Shoulder:
- ❏ Angry today about something that occured in the past.

Chow Down:
- ❏ To eat.

Close but no Cigar:
- ❏ To be very near and almost accomplish a goal, but fall short.

Cock and Bull Story:
- ❏ An unbelievable tale.

Come Hell Or High Water:
- ❏ Any difficult situation or obstacle.

Crack Someone Up:
- ❏ To make someone laugh.

Cross Your Fingers:
- ❏ To hope that something happens the way you want it to.

Cry Over Spilt Milk:
- ❏ When you complain about a loss from the past.

Cry Wolf:
- ❏ Intentionally raise a false alarm.

Cup Of Joe:
- ❏ A cup of coffee.

Curiosity Killed The Cat:
- ❏ Being Inquisitive can lead you into a dangerous situation.

Cut to the Chase:
- ❏ Leave out all the unnecessary details and just get to the point.

Dark Horse:

❑   One who was previously unknown and is now prominent.

Dead Ringer:

❑   100% identical. A duplicate.

Devil's Advocate:

❑   Someone who takes a position for the sake of argument without believing in that particular side of the arguement. It can also mean one who presents a counter argument for a position they do believe in, to another debater.

Don't count your chickens before they hatch:

Don't rely on it until your sure of it.

Don't Put All Your Eggs In One Basket:

Do not put all your resources in one possibility.

Down To The Wire:

❑   Something that ends at the last minute or last few seconds.

Drastic Times Call For Drastic Measures:

❑   When you are extremely desperate you need to take extremely desperate actions.

Drink like a fish:

❑   To drink very heavily.

Drive someone up the wall:

❑   To irritate and/or annoy very much.

Dropping Like Flies:

❑   A large number of people either falling ill or dying.

Dry Run:

❑   Rehearsal.

Cock and Bull Story:

❑   An unbelievable tale.

Feeding Frenzy:

❑   An aggressive attack on someone by a group.

Field Day:

❑   An enjoyable day or circumstance.

Finding Your Feet:

❑   To become more comfortable in whatever you are doing.

Finger lickin' good:

❑   A very tasty food or meal.

Fixed In Your Ways:

❑   Not willing or wanting to change from your normal way of doing something.

Flash In The Pan:

❑ Something that shows potential or looks promising in the beginning but fails to deliver anything in the end.

Flea Market:

❑ A swap meet. A place where people gather to buy and sell inexpensive goods.

Flesh and Blood:

❑ This idiom can mean living material of which people are made of, or it can refer to someone's family.

Flip the Bird:

❑ To raise your middle finger at someone.

Foam at the Mouth:

❑ To be enraged and show it.

Fools' Gold:

❑ Iron pyrites, a worthless rock that resembles real gold.

From Rags To Riches:

❑ To go from being very poor to being very wealthy.

Funny Farm:

❑ A mental institutional facility.

Get Down to Brass Tacks:

❑ To become serious about something.

Get Over It:

❑ To move beyond something that is bothering you.

Get Up On The Wrong Side Of The Bed:

❑ Someone who is having a horrible day.

Get Your Walking Papers:

❑ Get fired from a job.

Give Him The Slip:

❑ To get away from. To escape.

Go Down Like A Lead Balloon:

❑ To be received badly by an audience.

Go For Broke:

❑ To gamble everything you have.

Go Out On A Limb:

❑ Put yourself in a tough position in order to support someone/something.

Go The Extra Mile:

❑ Going above and beyond whatever is required for the task at hand.

Good Samaritan:

- ❑ Someone who helps others when they are in need, with no discussion for compensation, and no thought of a reward.

Great Minds Think Alike:

- ❑ Intelligent people think like each other.

Green Room:

- ❑ The waiting room, especially for those who are about to go on a tv or radio show.

Gut Feeling:

- ❑ A personal intuition you get, especially when feel something may not be right.

Haste Makes Waste:

- ❑ Quickly doing things results in a poor ending.

Hat Trick:

- ❑ When one player scores three goals in the same hockey game. This idiom can also mean three scores in any other sport, such as 3 homeruns, 3 touchdowns, 3 soccer goals, etc.

Have an Axe to Grind:

- ❑ To have a dispute with someone.

Head Over Heels:

- ❑ Very excited and/or joyful, especially when in love.

Hell in a Handbasket:

- ❑ Deteriorating and headed for complete disaster.

High Five:

- ❑ Slapping palms above each others heads as celebration gesture.

High on the Hog:

- ❑ Living in Luxury.

Hit The Books:

- ❑ To study, especially for a test or exam.

Hit The Hay:

- ❑ Go to bed or go to sleep.

Hit The Nail on the Head:

- ❑ Do something exactly right or say something exactly right.

Hit The Sack:

- ❑ Go to bed or go to sleep.

Hocus Pocus:

- ❑ In general, a term used in magic or trickery.

Hold Your Horses:

- ❑ Be patient.

Icing On The Cake:

❑ When you already have it good and get something on top of what you already have.

Idle Hands Are The Devil's Tools:

❑ You are more likely to get in trouble if you have nothing to do.

It's A Small World:

❑ You frequently see the same people in different places.

Its Anyone's Call:

❑ A competition where the outcome is difficult to judge or predict.

Section 2
Pronunciation

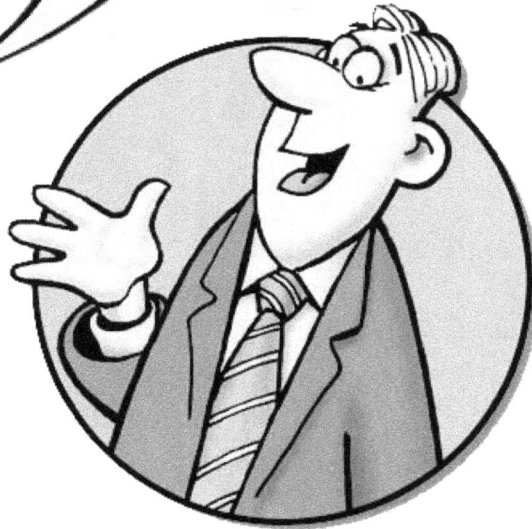

PRONUNCIATION

Speech sounds: we know that when we speak we produce a series of sounds and also that we produce different sounds in different combinations when we speak different languages. In order to understand how we communicate by speech and how speech works, it is necessary to study the sounds which make up speech and find out how these speech sounds are different from other sounds, how they are produced and how they can be identified, described and classified. An understanding of a nature of speech sounds in general will be helpful in studying the sounds of a specific language like English and in understanding how English speech works.

When we consider the sounds we hear around us, we notice that we produce and hear an amazing variety of sounds. We not only speak and hear others speak, but we also laugh, yawn, snore, cough, sneeze, shout with joy, or cry in pain or sorrow and play various musical instruments or hum tunes. But the important thing is that even in the midst of such a variety of different sounds, we know which of these sounds make up speech and which do not. In other words, we know whether someone is speaking or merely laughing, shouting or crying. This is so obvious that we don't even think about it. But it means that we have a mean of identifying and distinguishing speech sounds from all other types of sounds. We can do this not only when we know the language that is being spoken but even when we don't know the language. When we know the language, we recognize meaningful words in what we hear. When we don't know the language, we still perceive that the sounds we hear have certain features that help us to identify them as speech sounds, though we may not be able to recognize the words of the language. We may not consciously know what these features are, but use their presence to distinguish speech sounds from other sounds. In any study of the sounds of a language, be it English or any other, it is essential to identify these distinguishing features of speech sounds before we can identify, describe and classify the sounds of that particular language.

1. The most important distinguishing feature of speech sounds is that they can be separated and identified as distinct entities. For example, when we hear words like bus, tell or degree, we can identify the different sounds which make up each of them-/b/, and /s/ in bus, /t/, /e/ and /l/ in tell and /d/, /i/, /g/, /r/ and /i:/ in degree. But when we hear someone laughing or coughing, we cannot divide what we hear into constituent sounds because we cannot identify any separate entities that make up the sounds of laughing or coughing. A characteristic feature of language therefore is that it is made up of distinct sounds, which can be separated and differentiated from one another.

2. Dividing words into their constituent sounds shows another distinguishing feature of speech sounds. When we look at the sounds /b/, and /s/ separately, we notice that individual speech sounds do not have any meaning- /b/ does not mean anything nor do /s/ taken separately. But if we combine we have us, which also has meaning. Thus we can say that the distinct sounds that make up language do not have any meaning in themselves.

3. The distinct sounds that do not have any meaning in themselves acquire meaning when they are combined in specific ways. For example, if the sounds /t/, /e/ and /i/ which do not mean anything when taken separately are combined to form the sequences /te/ or /let/, they acquire meaning. But if we combine them to form /tle/, /lte/, /elt/ or /etl/, they do not have meaning. This is because /te/ and /let/ are words in English but /tle/, /lte/, /elt/ and /etl/ are not. Every language combines its sounds in different ways to form words with meaning and it is only when the sounds are combined in these ways that the combinations of sounds acquire meaning in that language.

4. Though individual sounds like /t/ or /e/ do not have any meaning in themselves, they have an important function in conveying meaning when they are combined with other sounds. If we consider the combinations /te/ and /bel/, for example, we see that both have meaning but different meanings. When they are combined with other sounds. If we consider the combinations /tel/ and /bel/, for example, we see that both have meaning but different meanings. What is that signals the difference in meaning between these two words? The only difference in sounds between the two words is that one has /t/ in the initial position whereas the other has /b/ in the same position. The other sounds are the same. We can therefore say that the sounds /t/ and /b/, though not having any meaning in themselves, signal a difference in meaning when they are combined with /el/. Similarly in /tel/ and /tu:l/, we find that the only difference between the two words is in the middle sounds /e/ and /u:/, whereas the initial and the final sounds are same. Here the sounds /e/ and /u:/ signal the difference in meaning between the words tell and tool. In /tel/ and /ten/, it is the final sounds /l/ and /n/, which are different the first two sounds in both the words being /t/ and /e/. The difference in meaning between the two words, tell and ten is, therefore, singnalled by /l/ and /n/. Thus individual sounds of language signal differences in meaning, though they do not have any meaning in themselves.

Speech sounds or sounds of language are distinguishable from other sounds because they have these four characteristic features, namely, a. they are distinct entities, b. they do not have any meaning in themselves, c. they convey meaning only when they are combined in specific ways and d. in specific combinations they signal contrasts in meaning.

Identification of Sounds

English like other languages has distinct set of sounds. Some of the sounds used in English may be found in other languages also. Examples are the initial sounds in words like pot, tin, keep, interest, egg and art. But there are other sounds in English that may not be found in other languages like the initial sounds in fool or zoo. Many Indian languages, for example do not have these sounds. Conversely, Indian languages have sounds like/l/ and /n/, which are nopt found in English. It is therefore necessary to identify the distinct sounds of every language separately.

In order to identify the sounds of a language, we make use of two of the distinctive features of speech sounds, one, they combine in specific way to form words. When the substitution of one sound by another in a word results in a new word with a different meaning, we take the two sounds to be distinct sounds of that language. Thus in the word pin, if we substitute the sound /b/ for /p/ in the initial position, we get a new word, bin and we can therefore conclude that /p/ and /b/ are distinct sounds of English. Similarly, /e/ and /i/, the middle sounds in the set and sit, can be identified as distinct sounds of English, since the substitution of one in the place of another results-in a different word. By repeating this process with a large number of words we arrive at the complete set of distinct sounds in English. For example, words like pin, bin, tin, kin, din, gin, thin, sin, shin, fin and chin have different sounds only in the initial position with the second and third sounds being identical in all of them, and therefore, we identify the initial sounds in these words as distinct sounds of English. Similarly, if we consider words like hit, hat, hut, heat, hurt, hot, hoot, heart, hate and height, we can identify the middle sounds in these words as distinct sounds of English. Using this procedure it has been found that there are 44 sounds in English; 20 of these are vowels and 24 consonants.

The distinct sounds of language are called phonemes. A phoneme is the minimal unit of sound in a language. The pairs of words in which the substitution of one sound by another helps us to identify the distinctive sounds of a language are called minimal pairs. A minimal pair is a pair of words that differ only in one sound. This sound, which marks the only difference between the two words, occurs in the same position in the two words, while the sounds in the other positions are the same. Some examples of minimal pairs in English are bat and mat, chip and ship, where the initial sounds are different; sum and sun, seat and seed, where the final sounds are different; and tan and tin, and pen and pun, where the middle sounds are different.

Right pronunciation is of great importance in spoken English. English is not a very phonetic language e.g. we do not speak exactly what is written. We don't confront such problems in Hindi or in our regional languages. They are phonetic. We read what we write. The situation becomes more complicated when different states and countries use their peculiar accent while speaking English. As a result, there is Indian English (Hinglish), Chinese English, Japanese English, American English, etc. Even in our own country, south Indians, north Indians, Bengalis, etc. speak English in different accents as influenced by their respective mother tongues.

A number of English words are not pronounced strictly in the same way. Most words have more than one pronunciation depending upon the factor like speed of speaking, background noise, speaker's accent, perception of the listener and also on how many times a word is repeated. We will therefore not overemphasise or be very strict with pronunciation norms. In this book, we explain the British way of pronunciation as spoken by the British Broadcasting Corporation (BBC), TV newsreaders without emphasis on American pronunciation. We shall be using a small set of symbols that represent various sounds. This principal of writing is known as *phonemic*.

You probably want to know what the purpose of this book is, and what you can expect to learn from it. An important purpose of the course is to explain how English is pronounced in the accent normally chosen as the standard for people learning the English spoken in England. Therefore this general information in the context of a general theory about speech sounds and how they are used in language; this theoretical context is called phonetics and phonology.

In any language we can identify a small number of regularly used sounds (vowels and consonants) that we call phonemes; for example, the vowels in the words 'pin' and 'pen' are different phonemes and so are the consonants at the beginning of the words 'pet' and 'bet'. Because of the notoriously confusing nature of English spelling it is particularly important to learn to think of English pronunciation in terms of phonemes rather than letters of the alphabet.

As most people know, we often use special symbols to represent speech sounds; a list of the symbols is given at the end of this chapter. Stress (which could be roughly described as the relative strength of a syllable) and intonation (the use of the pitch of the voice to convey meaning) are equally important.

One of the things that everybody knows about languages is that they have different accents. Languages are pronounced differently by people from different geographical places, from different social classes of different ages and different educational backgrounds. The word 'accent' is often confused with dialect. The accent that we concentrate on is the one that is recommended for foreign learns studying British English.

Received Pronunciation (usually abbreviated to its initials RP) is the most familiar accent used by most announcers and newsreaders on international BBC broadcasting channels.It would be an interesting exercise to identify the ways I which they differ from RP and even to learn some examples of different accent yourself.

Short Vowels:

Syllable is a unit of pronunciation with a vowel sound it may or may not contain a consonant. A syllable forms a word or part of word. Often long words are divided into two or three syllables. For example the word bedroom is divided into two syllables <u>bed</u> and <u>room</u>. The word 'bedroom' is not pronounced at a stretch. There in a very slight pause between <u>bed</u> and <u>room</u> represented as bedroom. (A dot is placed between two syllables)

Stress is the emphasis laid on a word syllable. Most long words in English are not pronounced on level tone. For example, The word 'academic' has three syllables aca.dem.ic since this words is pronounced with stress on the second syllable <u>demic</u> we shall write the first syllable <u>aca</u> which is not to be stressed in light print and second one which is to be stressed in bold print. Thus the word will appear as aca.dem.ic.

A List of Short Vowels

I	Big, b<u>u</u>sy, B<u>i</u>har
e	F<u>ea</u>ther, <u>n</u>eck, d<u>e</u>sk
æ	B<u>a</u>t, b<u>a</u>gg<u>a</u>ge, ch<u>a</u>t
ɒ	P<u>o</u>t, h<u>o</u>t, acr<u>o</u>ss
ʊ	P<u>u</u>ll, b<u>u</u>ll, b<u>oo</u>k

Short Vowels : Λ, I, e, æ, ɒ ʊ

A List of Long Vowels

i	B<u>ea</u>t, m<u>ea</u>w, p<u>ea</u>ce
ɜ	B<u>i</u>rd, f<u>e</u>rn, p<u>u</u>rse
a	C<u>a</u>rd, h<u>a</u>lf, p<u>a</u>ss
ɔ	B<u>oa</u>rd, t<u>o</u>rn, h<u>o</u>rse
u	F<u>oo</u>d, s<u>oo</u>n, l<u>oo</u>se

Diphthongs:

iə	Beard, law, fierce
eə	Aired, care, scare
ʊ ə	Moored, tour
eI	Paid, pair, face
aI	Tide, time, nice
ɔI	Void, toil, voice
əʊ	Load, home, most
aʊ	Loud, gown, house

RP has a large number of diphthong sounds which consist of a movement or glide from one vowel or another. A vowel which remains constant and does not glide is called a pure vowel and one of the most common pronunciation mistakes that result in the learner of English having a 'foreign' accent is the production of pure vowels where a <u>diphthong</u> should be pronounced. In terms of length, diphthong are like long vowels, the most important thing to remember about them is that the diphthongs first part is much longer and stronger than the second part.

Vowels

In English Grammar, there are five vowels *a, e, i, o, u*. They are pronounced in different ways when used in a word.

This letter is usually pronounced as (in weak form) when it comes in isolation before a consonant speeding knocked down this may be pronounced in a strong for i.e., if it is to be emphasised z. e. this is a (ei) problem but not the only one of its kind.

A

Words	Stressed and Non-stressed Syllables
Tap	Tæp
Tape	tæpe
car	keə
Care	ka:
Father	fa-thər
Swan	swän
Walk	Wŏk
Many	Man.y
Village	Vill.age
Necessary	Nec.e.ssary
Agree	

E

Words	Stressed and Non-stressed Syllables
Bed	Bəd
Eve	ev
Ever	Ev.er
Here	hir
There	ther
Were	wir
Very	Ver.i

I

Words	Stressed and Non-stressed Syllables
Ship	Ship
Pipe	PiP
High	hī
Fire	Fiər
Medicine	Med.Icine

The Larynx: The larynx has several very important functions in speech, when we breathe the air passes through the trachea and the larynx. The front of the larynx comes to the point and you feel this point at the front of your neck particularly if you are a man. Or slim. The point is commonly called the Adam's apple.

O

Words	Stressed and Non-stressed Syllables
Cod	käd
Code	köd
Copy	Cop.Y
Colour	Col.Our
Women	Wom.En
Woman	Wom.an
Observe	əb-zərv
Forget	fər-get

*Generally, r is not pronounced in **forget**.*

U

Words	Stressed and Non-stressed Syllables
Tub	təb
Bull	bul
Tube	tüb
Sugar	Sug.ar
Failure	Fai.lure
July	Juliə
mustache	məs-tash

Phonology: When we talk about how phonemes function in language, and the relationships among the different phonemes – when in other words, we study the abstract side of the sounds of language, we are studying a related but different subject that we call *phonology*.

B

Words	Stressed and Non-stressed Syllables
Bat	bæt
Ballet	bæl.et
Balled	bæl.əd
Bury	ber/.i, ber.i
Beer	biər
Bent	ben.t
Best	B~best
Bolt	bəʊlt, boʊlt
Boat	bəʊt, boʊt
Bow	baʊ, bəʊ

C

Words	Notes	Stressed and Non-stressed Syllables
Cell		Sel
Cycle	Before vowels e, i, and y, c is pronounced as s.	Si-kəl
Specify		Specif.ic

Social Vicious Ocean	In suffixes- <u>cial</u>, <u>cious</u>, <u>cient</u>andtheir derivatives <u>c</u> makes an<u>sh</u>sound.	So.cial Vicio.us o.cean
Succeed	When <u>c</u> is doubled it produces as <u>k</u> and <u>s</u> sound	sək-sēd
Nice		n īs
Occupy	Here one <u>c</u> is silent	Occu.py
Cat	In most cases <u>c</u> is pronounced as <u>k</u>	kat
Indict	Spoken as indict <u>c</u> is silent	in-dit

D

Words	Notes	Stressed and Non-stressed Syllables
Desk	Consonant- <u>d</u> is very consistent. It makes only one sound, that of <u>d</u> as in desk, bed	desk
Duck		dək
Wednesday	The letter <u>d</u> is not pronounced and <u>s</u> produces the sound of <u>z</u>	Wednes.day
Procedure	(The letter <u>r</u> super scripted) is very lightly pronounced as has been mentioned before also.	Proce.dure
Solider	Letter <u>d</u> is pronounced <u>j</u>	So.ldiar
Shaped	D can be pronounced as <u>t</u> in words like shaped, hoped, tipped.	shäpt

Nasals: The basic characteristic of a nasal consonant is that the air escapes through the nose. For this to happen, the soft palate must be lowered; in the case of all the other consonants, and all vowels the soft palate is raised and air cannot pass through the nose. In the nasal consonants, however the air does not pass through the mouth; it is prevented by a complete closure in the mouth at some point.

F

Words	Notes	Stressed and Non-stressed Syllables
Fit	Consonant f mostly produces f sound as in <u>fatoften</u> (<u>t</u> is mostly silent in this word)	fit
Cuff	When <u>f</u> is doubled one <u>f</u> is silent as it <u>off</u> also.	kəf
Of	<u>V</u> sound is produced misted of <u>f</u>	əv
Rough	<u>Gh</u> or <u>ph</u>at the or beginning produce the sound <u>f</u> as in (phone)	rəf

G

Words	Notes	Stressed and Non-stressed Syllables
Gem	There are two pronunciation of gz.e. g as d3	jem
Age		
	Or j and g as in give, go, gate etc.	aj
Geol.	Pronounced as jail.	Jəil
Gnat	G is often silent before n.	nät
Go		gö

Symbols: symbols are for one of two purposes; either they are symbols for phonemes (phonemic or phoneme symbols) or they are phonetic symbols. The most important point to remember is the rather obvious seeming fact that the number of phonemic symbols must be exactly the same as the number of phonemes we decide exist in the language.

H

Words	Notes	Stressed and Non-stressed Syllables
Head	The usual pronunciation of this latter is h	hed
Oh	H is silent here.	ōh
Rhythm	H is also silent following r.	Rh.yth.m
Heir	In words like heir, honest honor and hour, the initial h is silent. E.g. word heir in pronounced as air with little stress over r.	er

J

Words	Notes	Stressed and Non-stressed Syllables
Jam	The consonantJ is usually	Jam
Raj	Pronounced as d3 or j as in jump	räJ

The Syllable: The syllable is a very important unit. Most people seem to believe that, even if they cannot define what a syllable is, they can count how many syllables there are in a given word or sentence. If they are asked to do this they often tap their finger as they count, which illustrates the syllable's importance in the rhythm of speech. As a matter of fact, if one tries the experiment of asking English speakers to count the syllables in, say, a tape-recorded sentence, there is often a considerable amount of disagreement.

K

Words	Notes	Stressed and Non-stressed Syllables
Kate	The letter k is pronounced k in general as in kite, kate, kid, key.	Kat
Khaki	In this word letter h is not pronounced. So we should say kaki.	Kha.ki
Knack	In words beginning with kn, k is usually silent as in knit, know etc.	nak

L

Words	Notes	Stressed and Non-stressed Syllables
Like	In general letter l is pronounced as l as in lamb, life, leg etc.	lik
Calf		kaf
calm	L is silent when it comes before letter f, m and k as in yolk.	käm
Could		kəd
would	In letter ould of model verb like could and would, l is silent.	wəd

Strong and weak syllables: one of the most noticeable features of English is that many syllables are weak; this is true of many other languages. We could describe them partly in terms of stress as the strong syllables are stressed and weak syllables unstressed.

M

Words	Notes	Stressed and Non-stressed Syllables
Mother	The letter m is always spoken as m	Moth.er
Hymn		him
Condemn	In the letters mn coming at the end. N is silent	Con.demn

N

Words	Notes	Stressed and Non-stressed Syllables
Nail		nal
mine	The use of letter n is very consistent as it usually makes only n sound	mïn
Anxious		Anx. ous
bank	Letter x is pronounced as k and n is pronounced as (ng sound).	band

Rhythm: The notion of rhythm involves some noticeable event happening at regular intervals of time; one can detect the rhythm of a heart-beat of a flashing light or of a piece of music. It has often been claimed that English speech is rhythmical, and that the rhythm is detectable in the regular occurrence of stressed syllables; of course, it is not suggested that the timing as regular as clock- the regularity of occurrence is only relative.

P

Words	Notes	Stressed and Non-stressed Syllables
Pen	Letter p is mostly spoken as p as in tap, top, ape etc.	pen
Pneumatic	P can be silent in the combinations.	Penumat.k
Psalm	Of ph,ps and pt. L is silent in the word psalm.	säm
Receipt	The word should be spoken as (----)	ri-set
Corps	To be pronounced as kor with little stream on letter r.	kor
Cupboard	Letter p is silent in both the distances. This word should be pronounced as kuberd.	Cupb.oard
Raspberry	The pronunciation should be raazberi.	Rasp.berry
Supper	Where p is doubled as in dipper one p is silent.	Supp.er

Q

Words	Notes	Stressed and Non-stressed Syllables
Queen	Generally q is followed by u and pronounced as kw or k	kwew
antique		

R

Words	Notes	Stressed and Non-stressed Syllables
Red	In British English r is pronounced.	red
Bore	Only when it appears before vowels. Also it is sound only before vowels.	bor
Car	In the word car, r is very lightly stressed in US English r is fully spoken.	kär

S

Words	Notes	Stressed and Non-stressed Syllables
Sack	Mostly the s sound in this consonant is very consonant. However it is pronounced in other ways also.	sak
Case	In other ways also.	kad
Rise	Z is a common pronunciation of the letter s.	riz

Asia ä-zhe-ä Tension Station Persuasion	In suffixes like <u>sion</u>, <u>sure</u>, <u>sia</u> and their derivatives <u>s</u> is spoken as or 3	Ten.sion Sta.tion Persua.sion
Treasure		Treasu.re
Psychology	Letter <u>p</u> is silent here.	Psycholo.gy
Circus circle	The first letter c is pronounced as <u>s</u> and the second one as <u>k</u>	Cir.cle
Debris	Letter s is silent in this French <u>word</u>.	De.bri

T

Words	Notes	Stressed and Non-stressed Syllables
Get Tap Butter Castle	The letter t has constant pronunciation is the beginning and at the end of a word. However it has other sounds also. When appearing between two vowels. One t is silent. T is also silent in many words carried from French. The following words are.	git tap b.ə-tər ka-səl
Depot	Pronounced askasel, depo.	di-po
Ballet	Bele and buke.	ba-la
Bouquet		bo ka
Negotiate Affection station	A common pronunciation of t is (sh) where it is followed by a suffix which begins with letter I	Nego.tiate Offec.tion Sta.tion
Adventure Picture	The letter t is also spoken ts (ch)	Adven.ture Picture
Listen	T is silent when it is followed by s or f as in often	List.en

V

Words	Notes	Stressed and Non-stressed Syllables
Van	The consonant <u>v</u> is always pronounced as <u>v</u> as in van and love.	Van
Volkswagen	In this word from German language, pronunciation starts with <u>f</u>.	Volkswa.gen

w

Words	Notes	Stressed and Non-stressed Syllables
Wet	This consonant is most often spoken as w as in wit, wet, swing, away etc.	Wet
Now		nav
Write	In the spelling combination of wr , w is not pronounced	rit
Two	W is also silent in some instances when tw come in the beginning.	tu
Answer	In some words where sw is in middle w is silent.	An.swer

Special note: Initial hers wh are pronounced as w in words like, when, why, what, where. So these should be respectively spoken as wen, wai, wot and ware.

X

Words	Notes	Stressed and Non-stressed Syllables
Box	This letter rarely occurs at the beginning. It is pronounced as ks as in box.	baks
Examine	Here x is pronounced as a combination of g2	Exam.in
Noxious	In this word x is pronounced as ks or ksh	Nox. ious
Xylophone	When the letter x comes at the beginning it is usually pronounced as z	Xy.lo.phone
x-ray	Another pronunciation of x is eks	eks-ra
Exclaim	Here x is pronounced as ksk	ika-klam
Exceed	Before the vowel letter I or e it is pronounced as ks.	iksed
Luxury	Here x is pronounced as kzh	Lux.ry

Y

Words	Notes	Stressed and Non-stressed Syllables
Youth	This letter can act both as vowel and consonant. At the beginning, it occurs as a vowel producing the sound of j.	yu
Yes		yes
Myth	Acting as a vowel y here has a short pronunciation of I as also in nymph.	mith
Fly	It has a long pronunciation of a	fli
Study	If the word ends with y a short I is used as study and lady	Stud.y

Z

Words	Notes	Stressed and Non-stressed Syllables
Zest		zest
Gaze		gaz
Zero	The consonant z is mostly spoken a z as in zest, gaze, zero.	Ze.ro
Seizure	When followed by letter u, it can be pronounced as 3	sei-zure
Rendezvous	This is a word borrowed from French. Z is silent here. It should be spoken as rondivoo	Ren.dez.vous
Scissors	Here ss consonants are spoken a z lettersz are also pronounced z as in czar. Actually in words like was, rags, does, rose etc. the letter s is usually pronounced as z	Sciss.ors

Some of the Phonetic Symbols are as follows:

Phonetics or pronunciation is a matter of understanding sounds and using them properly in our speech. To use certain words constantly and continuously is the key to learning any language and English is no exception.

Iː READ	I SIT	ʊ BOOK	uː TOO	Iə HERE	eI DAY	John & Sarah Free Materials 1996
e MEN	ə AMERICA	ɜː WORD	ɔː SORT	ʊə TOUR	ɔI BOY	əʊ GO
æ CAT	ʌ BUT	ɑː PART	ɒ NOT	eə WEAR	ɑI MY	ɑʊ HOW
p PIG	b BED	t TIME	d DO	tʃ CHURCH	dʒ JUDGE	k KILO	g GO
f FIVE	v VERY	θ THINK	ð THE	s SIX	z ZOO	ʃ SHORT	ʒ CASUAL
m MILK	n NO	ŋ SING	h HELLO	l LIVE	r READ	w WINDOW	j YES

Note: Phonetics & Pronunciation is an indispensables part of learning this vast and complex language. Basically, phonetic symbols are a great help when it comes to learning to pronounce English words correctly. As you open any English/Dictionary, you can easily find the correct pronunciation of words, you don't know by reading/deciphering the phonetic symbol (alphabet)/written next to the words.

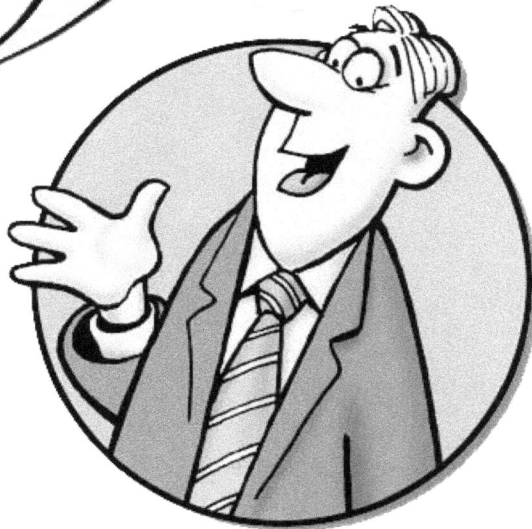

Section 3
Conversation

CONVERSATION

The art of conversation like any art is a skill of elegance, nuance and creative execution.

Without flair and panache, most things become drudgery. Why settle for drudgery when you can have art?

When it comes to the art of conversation we've all met people who seem to have knack for it. They can talk to anybody about anything and they seem to do it with complete ease. And while it's true that there are those who are born with the gift of gab, luckily for the rest of us, conversation skills can be developed and mastered.

In my article Good Communication Skills - Key to Any Success, I talk about the importance of being a good communicator and I give tips on how to convey ideas and information successfully. Many of the same tips hold true for developing good conversational skills. Have a look at the article for added tips which I won't be repeating here.

Conversation is a form of communication; however, it is usually more spontaneous and less formal. We enter conversations for purposes of pleasant engagement, in order to meet new people, to find out information, and to enjoy social interactions. As far as types of conversation, they vary anywhere from intellectual conversations and information exchanges to friendly debate and witty banter.

While there is more to having good conversation skills than being a comedian, dramatic actor, or a great story teller, it is not necessary to become more gregarious, animated, or outgoing. Instead, you can develop the ability to listen attentively, ask fitting questions, and pay attention to the answers - all qualities essential to the art of conversation. With diligent practice and several good pointers, anyone can improve their conversation skills.

Tips on How to Improve Your Conversational Skills

Show interest and be curious. People who are genuinely interested in others are usually interesting themselves. Why? Because they are more open to learning about and understanding new things. Showing interest also encourages the other person to be relaxed and share information more freely. Display attentiveness by keeping good eye contact and listening actively.

If you happen to be shy and need time to warm up before you share your own views, you can ask open-ended questions or encourage the other person to elaborate on their insights. This kick-starts the conversation and before you know it you are engaged in a good conversational flow.

Ensure there is a balance of give and take. A conversation can get boring quickly if one person is doing all the talking while the other is trying to get a word in edgewise. When that happens whoever is not talking begins to tune out and there is no conversation!

There can be many reasons for a lack of give and take. Sometimes nervousness can get in the way and you ramble on without realizing it. Or, nervousness can make you freeze and you don't know what to say next. If you find yourself freezing up, take a deep breath and do your best to focus; smile, and then reflect on what you want to say. If the other person is the rambler and you've tried several times to interject but haven't been able to, then excuse yourself politely and move on.

If later on you realize that you were the rambler (heaven forbid), then at least you will have made the most important step towards improvement which is - awareness.

Determine whether your tendency to dominate a conversation is due to nervousness or self-involvement. Either way, review the conversation in your head. Look for spots where you could have paused and allowed the other person to talk. For future conversations a good rule of thumb is after you make a point, pause for either agreement or an alternative point of view. Observe body language for cues whether to stop or continue. For example, is the person glossy-eyed and therefore bored? Are they moving towards you to speak and you just keep on talking? Are they looking elsewhere (for an escape) while you are carrying on? In a good conversation each person needs to express themselves or it is no longer a conversation but a monologue.

Be interesting and have something to say. While you don't have to be a comedian, entertainer, or brilliant raconteur, you do need to be interesting otherwise what would you say? If you are not well informed, tend not to read much, or have very few interests, you will have very little to talk about except yourself. Unfortunately, no one wants to hear about your latest troubles, conquests, or daily routine. Yet so many dull conversationalists believe that's what people want to hear from them. Who hasn't been stuck with someone at a social event who blathers away about their family history, latest job interview, or the like?

To avoid being that person, become knowledgeable about world events, people in the news, or what's going on locally. Take time to keep up with the latest music, new technological discoveries, or recent best sellers. No one can know everything, so if you can enlighten someone during the course of a conversation, you'll be a hit! By the same token, you can learn something new as well.

Of course, not all conversations are knowledge sharing gatherings or discussions of global import. Many, especially at social functions, consist of light-hearted and cheerful banter. In such cases, be aware of the tone and mood of the conversation and go with the flow. If you are not particularly good at one-liners, or much of a jokester, you can always listen, smile and enjoy the humor. Never act like you feel out of place or ill at ease.

Be relaxed, be yourself. If you are on edge, or trying to be someone you're not, it will show and therefore doom a conversation to failure before it starts. Admittedly, if you are not relaxed it's hard to appear as if you are. Slow down and take a deep breath. If you don't do your best to relax, you will end up saying something silly, unintelligible, or unrelated to the conversation. Also smile warmly; it will make you appear pleasant and therefore more approachable. Worth noting: if you are trying to hard to be something you're not, you will come across as a fake or a wannabe.

To start a conversation, go up to someone and introduce yourself. It is both polite and necessary to start things off smoothly. If the occasion calls for it, you can offer a handshake and then smile and make eye contact. Being friendly puts the other person at ease and opens the door for them to introduce themselves. If, for whatever reason, your attempt is not well-received and you notice the other person is cool or standoffish, bow out gracefully and move on. Do not take it as a rejection; merely consider that the person has their reasons for not reciprocating. Perhaps they are not feeling well, have had a bad day, or are not in the mood for conversation.

To improve, practice and then practice some more. The art of conversation, like any skill, takes practice. Do not expect to be adept after your first few attempts. It will take practice as well as exposure to many different social situations. A good way to get practice before you venture out to an event is with family members and people you are comfortable with. They can give you helpful and supportive feedback, which in turn gives you something to work on. You can never have too much practice!

Quick-Tips for the Art of Conversation

- ❑ Do not dominate a conversation or make it all about you. A monologue is not conversation.
- ❑ Show interest and curiosity in others.
- ❑ Strive for a balance of give and take.
- ❑ Be an active listener by maintaining good eye contact and asking pertinent questions.
- ❑ Train yourself to relax by using visualization, meditation, or other relaxation methods. Being relaxed is vital for good conversation.
- ❑ Do not interrupt and cut in with your own ideas before the other person is finished speaking.
- ❑ Maintain an open mind; everyone has a right to express themselves even if you don't agree with what they are saying.
- ❑ Although this is cliché, try to avoid topics such as sex, religion and politics. You would be surprised at how many people get trapped by them and end up in verbal battle, not conversation.
- ❑ Be prepared by staying on top of the latest news, developments and world events.
- ❑ Be approachable by staying relaxed, smiling and maintaining a friendly attitude.
- ❑ Possessing the art of conversation improves personal, social and work relationships. It gives you the opportunity to meet interesting new people and introduces you to various new topics and subject matter. With practice and application anyone can improve their conversation skills.

Why You Need To Directly Practise Your Social Skills

To improve your social skills you have to practice them. That sentence is probably one of the most important ones on this site. All the advice on this site can help you have a better idea of what to do or not to do, but you still have to hone the actual skills in real life. It's the same for any other ability people can have. This point is really basic, and you can read the same advice in dozens of other places. I still have to mention it though because it's so important.

If your interpersonal skills are a little shabby, you've likely spent much less time socializing compared to most people. Some combination of your personality and your life experiences has caused you to miss out and fall behind your peers. You need to get out there as much as you can and put in the hours to catch up. You need time to become familiar with all the little things everyone else learned years ago.

You have to try out all the different aspects of interacting with people, make your inevitable mistakes, and slowly get the hang of things. With practice, situations that you used to awkwardly bumble your way through will turn into ones you've come across dozens of times, and which you know how to handle. Skills and traits that feel forced and stilted at first will become second nature, and almost feel like you've always had them. You'll start to gain a confidence that comes from realizing you've been around people successfully before, and you can do it again.

Learning by Observation is Also Important

You have to directly practice skills like making conversation. While you're around people, you also can't help but take in what everyone is else doing and incorporate some of the ideas you pick up into yourself. This goes for learning positive new things to do, but also what to avoid. It's good to be open to learning from anyone. Sometimes you may not be crazy about a person on the whole, but you could still pick up some good isolated skills from them.

Like with direct practice, this process is gradual. You won't change overnight just from watching people, but eventually the benefits will pile up. It's another reason to simply spend more time in social situations. At times the observation process is conscious and deliberate, like you'll notice someone has an effective way of introducing themselves, and decide to do the same thing. Just as often, it all happens automatically. As you hang around people enough, certain traits of theirs will rub off on you without you noticing it's happening.

Attitudes have to be Practised As Well

Your social success will partially be determined by your attitudes; how confident you are, how positive your self-image is, how optimistic you are, how you view other people, and so on. Helpful attitudes have to be built up over time too. They're quite abstract and psychological, but they still have to be earned through real-world experiences and successes that support feeling that way.

Practising Specifically What You Want to Work On vs. Spillover Effects

A point on what types of practice experiences to seek out: There are lots of different ways to socialize with other people. Chatting to someone over coffee isn't the same as debating them. In one sense, you'll get good specifically at what you practice. Learning to have deep conversations with people won't make you all that much better at cracking jokes and being the life of a party. If you want to get better at something in particular, like being able to think of things to say in group conversations, then put yourself in more situations where you can do that.

Sometimes someone will take up an activity like public speaking, hoping it will help them get along with people more easily, and then later find that the skills needed to give good speeches don't 100% translate into helping them chat to people at social gatherings. One is rehearsed and pre-planned; the other is more improvised and spontaneous.

So on one hand; try to directly work on the things you want to get better at. But it's obviously not that cut and dry. Getting better at one type of socializing can have spillover effects into other areas. To get back to the example from a second ago, becoming a good speaker may make you more confident and polished on the whole. Your sense of humor, or ability to tell a good story may improve. Learning to handle the nerves from speaking before a crowd may make you more at ease in smaller groups. Realistically you'll end up doing a mix of specific and indirect practice. It all helps in the long run.

Good Conversation is one of Life's Pleasures

Some people are better conversationalists than others. What skills or techniques do they employ? Stan James and I have been interested in this question for a long time and first discussed it in Costa Rica last summer. We came up with a grab bag of do's and don'ts for in-person conversations (not email or phone). Your additions?

Don't selfishly hijack. This is the most annoying habit of bad conversationalists. You say, "I met some really interesting people at that conference." He says, "Really? I met nobody interesting." Or, you say, "My classes are all terrific." She says, "Really? Mine suck." In other words, whatever you say he takes as an invitation to share his personal experience / opinion instead of probing on your statement or at least clarifying or re-phrasing it. Once you start watching for this you see it all the time. Don't be that guy. Don't hijack conversations to bring it back to yourself. Wait your turn. Be interested in the other person.

Answer questions at the appropriate level of detail. If you're in a job interview and the potential employer asks about your last job, you will offer detail. If you're at a cocktail party and someone you don't know asks the same question, the appropriate (initial) answer calls for very little detail. Too many people deploy the same answer to common questions without customizing it to the particular conversation.

In groups, avoid topics that not all can follow. Pursue topics common to all participants.

Don't try too long to remember something. To use a technical term, "time-out" after 10 seconds. Don't make everyone wait as you try to remember the name of that book you were reading ("Gosh what was its name, I know it, it's, it's, it's, gosh let me think…"). Drop it and move on. It will come to you later.

Fidelity to an objective isn't always necessary. Some business meetings call for strict adherence to an agenda. But many of the best conversations follow new and unknown directions. The joy is in the journey.

Be self-aware about self-interruptions. Meanderings and tangents contribute to the wonderful spontaneity of conversations. Just announce your intention to pursue an off-point before doing so. E.g., "Ok, I want to come back to this, but let me tell you a quick related story…"

Feel free to shift gears quickly. After you've plumbed the depths of a topic, move on, even if it's abrupt. Not every new statement needs to iteratively build on the prior one. For example, you talk about business ideas with your conversation partner, there's a pause, and then you say, "Ok, changing topics, how's your family?"

Recognize "just need to be heard" conversations. These are unique conversations between friends or romantic partners. One party just wants to feel heard, not engage in debate or discussion. The best thing you can do is listen really well. E.g., she says, "I feel like nobody at work appreciates me. I'm there ten hours a day and I hardly ever get a thank-you." You say, "Yeah. So you're saying nobody at the office is giving you love?"

The Traffic Light 'rule' of communication. "During the first 30 seconds of an utterance, your light is green. That means your listener is listening and not thinking you talk too much. During the next 30 seconds, your light is yellow. That means the risk is increasing that your listener is bored, overwhelmed, or dying to respond. After the one-minute mark, your light is red. Yes, occasionally, you can go beyond a minute, for example, when telling an interesting story, but generally you should stop or ask a question."

Be okay with silence. Don't rush to fill silence in a conversation. Some people particularly need silent time to think and reflect, if only for a moment. And wasn't it Aristotle who said that true friendship is when silence between two people is comfortable?

Recognize people who are "getting in line" in the conversation. Notice people who tried to say something but got cut off. Notice people "raising their hand" to speak but haven't been able to say their two cents. Circle back to them.

Taking notes during the conversation. I've blogged about the pros and cons of taking notes during a one-on-one conversation. Pros: you remember what was talked about and show respect for the other person's ideas. Cons: can overly formalize the interaction and create a weird status dynamic if only one person is scribbling.

Don't deploy conversation-stopping phrases. "It's complicated" or "But here's a counterexample!" or "Correlation doesn't equal causation!"

Tell stories. Communication experts the world over agree that stories are the most effective way to convey ideas. Here are some tips on how to tell a good story.

Listen well. Listening skills deserves a post of its own. Suffice to say here that being an active, respectful, genuine listener will energize your conversation partner(s), and lead to a higher overall quality conversation. One way to improve on this front is to talk with good listeners (you know who they are because when you talk to them you feel heard). Notice their habits.

Recognize when the conversation is over. If you start talking about the stuff you started off with, it's sign you're looking back and nearing the end. If your partner seems to be disengaging (for example his eyes start wandering), take this as a cue. In any event, respect everyone's time and proactively bring a conversation to a close by saying, "This has been lots of fun. We should probably get going. But I really enjoyed it – thanks."

The need for good communication is imperative since we have to pass on the message that we want others to understand and immediately respond. Effective communication is possible only with the comprehensive knowledge of the language and its proper usage. With a number of examples given, it would become simpler and easier to understand different scenarios and communicate accordingly.

CHAPTER 1

BUYING A GIFT

Buying a gift is important and happens to us sometime or the other and therefore requires a good communication skill if we are looking for something specifically.

Salesman:	"Hello sir! May I help you?"
Customer:	Indeed you may. I'm looking for a birthday present for my daughter.
Salesman:	Very well sir, would you go for some wearing material like jeans, tops, shorts, Bermudas?
Customer:	Oh no! She is a grown up one and has lots of clothes. Besides, I'm not sure my choice will exactly match hers. What about that watch?
Salesman:	It is Rado, the American watch.
Customer:	Looks good. But then there are other watches like Omega, Cartier.
Salesman:	Well. They are costly ones. What is your budget?

You have these Japanese ones, Seiko, Casio etc.

Salesman:	Well, exactly speaking sir, it is not a watch shop. So we have selected items. Why don't you have a look as this wall Clock? There is a Cuckoo bird also which announces hours. Children will be quite fascinated by it. You have grand children?
Customer:	Yes, Thank you. May be they will welcome it. Is there anything else?
Salesman:	There is Chinese Ming vase (laughs). Of course it is an imitation but a very clever and beautiful one. Have a look at it.
Customer:	You're right, it looks very attractive.
Salesman:	You'll excuse me sir.

There is a bit of crowd. You can call me when you have made a choice if you fancy paintings. There is a piece hanging over there it is quite attractive. There is a price tag attached to every item. You can take your pick.

Customer:	A moment pleases, I think I have made my choice, the price also suits me. Will you please pack that vase for me?
Salesman:	Sure sir. Thank you.

CHAPTER 12

TALK ON METRO PLATFORM

When we meet people who are strangers and yet need to hit a conversation with them then the ability to communicate comes to the forefront and here we need to be polite courteous and distant at the same time.

Two people are standing on platform waiting for the train. One passenger talks to another standing nearby). Will the train to Karol Bagh arrive at this platform?

Second:	Yes.
First:	How much time will it take? Will it arrive shortly?
Second:	in three minutes, you can see it on the display board over there.
First:	I hope it wait be late.
Second:	That is rare. Are you travelling for the first time?
First:	Yes I'm rather nervous. It all looks so complicated. I had to ask for everything. At the ticket window it was a long queue and there was problem of change also.
Second:	Initially even I had problems but one gets the hang of it over a period of time. Well. The train is coming. Get ready. Be careful, don't go too near the track, and stand behind the yellow line.
First:	Thanks, by the way where are you going?
Second:	Same destination, Karol Bagh.
First:	Fine then we can be together.
Second:	There now. The train is stopping. Watch your step. Ah! Lucy we are there are two seats vacant
First:	I have travelled in Mumbai local also, but they are not even a match for Delhi metro. It is almost the same in Kolkata. Delhi metro is by far the best.
First:	I'm going to like it. It is so cool, calm and clean here. It is a noiseless train. Besides, they are clearly announcing all the coming stations and also which side the doors will open.
Second:	Yes, if you find a seat vacant, you can really relax. I wish they add more coaches on busy routes. They have already added an extra coach for ladies only.
First:	I'm glad about the ladies extra coach. My wife becomes nervous in a crowd. Karol bagh is approaching. I have found the journey delightful. Well. Thanks for your help and company.
Second:	You are welcome.

SCENE AT A BUS STAND

The 'bus stop' of a public transport point is important hub's where we come across the entire cross section of our society

Man:	(to the clerk at the window). Could you please tell me from where to buy ticket for Ajmer? There are no clear directions anywhere.
Another man:	He is too busy to answer. Come I'll tell you.
	First man; are you also going there?
Second man:	Yes. My name is Fateh khan.
First man:	I am kailash Gupta. Glad to meet you.
Khan:	Same here. Let's go to the ticket window. It is over there. Do you see that long queue?
Kailash:	Yes, it is going to take time.
Khan:	What is the use of <u>both</u> of us standing in the queue? If you want you can sit over there on the bench. I'll buy two tickets for Ajmer.
Kailash:	Oh! Thank you. I really need some rest. Here, please take the ticket money.
Khan:	You can go and relax. (At the ticket window) How much for two tickets for Ajmer?
Clerk:	Four hundred and thirty.
Khan:	Here is the money, please give me two tickets (to kailash) I have bought tickets, let us go and sit in the bus.
Kailash:	Thanks for tickets. This is the I.S.B.T stand, can you see the crowd and confusion around here.
Khan:	(to a man) Can you tell us where we will find the bus for Ajmer?
Man:	You could have asked at the ticket window itself. I'm also new here. Do you see that collie type of fellow over there? May be he will tell you.
Khan:	Thanks. Hello, there! Can you tell us where to find the bus for Ajmer?
Man:	Cross from over there. Be careful of the moving buses. You'll find the bus where number 10 is written.
Khan:	Thanks come Kailashji. Let's cross carefully.
(In the bus)	
Kailash:	If I am not mistaken you must be going to the Ajmer Sharif Dargah.
Khan:	Yes, and you?
Kailash:	I'm headed for the sacred pond Pushkar. But I'll visit the Dargah also. Almost all people who came here, visit Ajmer Sharif Dargah.
Kailash:	Be it so I'm very thankful to you khan sahib. Although a stranger you have helped me a lot. You are a very caring kind of person.
Khan:	Thanks. If you help others God will help you, it is as simple as that.

Chapter 4

TELESHOPPING

Television as a medium of buying and its impact on our ability to sort out our requirement the quick and easy way.

(A couple is watching a teleshopping programme at home.)

Anita:	What a beautiful necklace, Rahul .The price is Rs.1,998. They are also offering a free bangle set, earrings and that fancy wrist band.
Rahul:	Do you like them? I don't know much about these women things. If you fancy them, you can buy them. I have no objection. They rather look good to me also.
Anita:	Well the offer is for today only. Will you read the phone number for me, Rahul?
Rahul:	Well, The Delhi number is 011-22348567 one moment Anita. Do you think they will be as good as they look on the screen?
Anita:	Don't worry Rahul. These people are reliable. Many of my friends have purchased jewellery items from them and so far there have been no complaints.
Rahul:	Ok. Go ahead then.
Anita:	(rings) Hello! Well I'm speaking from Delhi. My name is Anita and right now I'm seeing your home shopping programme. It's a necklace and some other items.
Salesman:	(from other end) yes, ma'm. I have the programme displayed before me as well. Would you like to place an order?
Anita:	Yes, please.
Salesman:	I have your name phone number. Please tell me your postal address and also the item code number.
Anita:	Hold on for a moment. Where is the item code number?
Salesman:	Please look carefully at the left corner of the screen. The words are clearly displayed there as item code number.
Anita:	Yes, yes I see them. Please write the number it is 3489.
Salesman:	Thanks, and your address please.
Anita:	(tells the address) Please note down my landline number also. It is 24367892.
Salesman:	Thanks. We shall make the delivery within Seven days.
Anita:	Alright, and the payment?
Salesman:	As soon as you get, the delivery. Kindly pay the amount of Rs.1998, to the delivery man. Please keep the receipt carefully.

Anita: Ok but what if there is a complaint. You know we can pick and choose at a shop and even ask for replacement of a defective piece.

Salesman: Please don't worry. We are an internationally reputed firm. Such things don't happen with us. But should you have any complaint kindly ring me up. My name is Rawat. I'll immediately attend to you.

Anita: Thanks, we'll waiting for the delivery.

CHAPTER 5

A VISIT TO BIG BAZAAR

The bazaar or market place where trade takes place which is noisy and haphazard yet interesting, captivating, colourful and interactive.

(A husband and wife come across an advertisement in the newspaper regarding exchange of old things for new. They load their things in their car and reach big bazaar.)

Rajiv:	(to the guard at entrance) We have to exchange our old things for new. Which way to go?
Guard:	Please go straight and then left you'll find the place.
Rajiv:	Thanks.
An attendant:	(as they reach the place) Please park your car here.
Rajiv:	But then how shall we carry our goods? The exchange counter looks far away.
Attendant:	Don't worry sir. We'll help you.
	(They reach the spot)
Wife Sunita:	What an odd variety of things people have brought here. I wish we had brought our old fridge too.
Rajiv:	You're right. It consumes a lot of electricity besides being broken at places. But then there was no room in the car. Look that guy is bringing our things. I'm going to be with him so that our things are not misplaced. You keep standing here; we'll dump all our things here.
	(within an hour their things are valued and they are given purchase coupons)
Sunita:	Now for shopping. I'm glad we' had a heavy breakfast because it is going to take time here.
Rajiv:	(to an employee) could you please tell me which doors to enter, we want to make purchases.
Employee:	The middle one. You see a lot of people are entering from there.
Rajiv:	Right, Thank you.
Sunita:	(inside) Oh! What a big palace and so many items! It seems to have three or four floors. (To a salesman) Where is the kitchen section?
Salesman:	You'll find it on the right hand side madam. There are sign boards all over the palace.
Rajiv:	Sunita I going to look for washing machine and fridge. Don't get lost. When you're finished reach the electronic goods section.
A salesman:	May I help you sir? What are you looking for?

Rajiv:	Washing machine & Fridge.
Salesman:	Right sir, come with me. Here you are. (To another salesman) Show some washing machine and fridge to sir.
The other salesman:	This koryo washing machine from Korea is with a 5kg capacity. Look sir how sturdily it is build. It has two lids. The price is only 5000/- . (Further explains about the machine)
Rajiv:	It seems good to me. I'll buy it. Is the payment to be made here?
Salesman:	No sir. Please tell me your name, home address and phone number. Do you see that payment counter there? The machine will be packed and sent there. Also with this machine there is a free room heater.
Rajiv:	Thanks.
Sunita:	(to the salesman in kitchen section) How much is this frying pan?
Salesman:	(shows him the piece) It is only Rs700. It's a good quality non stick and....
Sunita:	What about this dinner set?
Salesman:	Please feel free to check and select them. All items have price tags attached to them. If you need any help. Call me.
Sunita:	(makes some purchases) Well I have selected these ones. What now?
Salesman:	Please tell me your name etc. Everything is computerized here. Reach that cash counter over there and you'll find your goods.
Sunita:	Thanks (meets Rajiv at the counter) what have you bought?
Rajiv:	Only a washing machine. Fridge maybe next time we can buy.
Counterman:	What is you and your wife's name sir? I'm typing out the receipts. Well! You have purchases worth Rs 8000/-. If you buy for two thousand rupees more of goods, you'll be given ten percent discount. It's a good opportunity.
Rajiv:	Thanks, but some other time.
Counterman:	Here is a book to keep reward of your purchases in future so that you can get a discount. Please bring it with you when you come next. Today's entries have been made. Here is your bill.
Rajiv:	Why this sales tax?
Counterman:	Well, it has to be paid. Some shops include it in the selling price. But we don't. One thing more sir, here is a lucky coupon. Ring me this Friday. You may win something even a car. (Smiles)
Rajiv:	(smiles) Thanks, here is the money. By the way can we pay with credit card also?
Counterman:	Of course you can. Actually a lot of people prefer that mode of payment.
	(Rajiv and Sunita collect their purchases the washing machine is being carried on a trolley by an attendant. There are checked by a guard at the exit gate and having their things placed in their car, they leave for home.)

CHILDREN'S BIRTHDAY PARTY

A sociological need to connect with people and this need has to be dealt with style and positive interaction.

(It is evening. The party has begun; some children are accompanied by their parents or grandparents.)

Sandeep: Welcome Mr. Khanna. I'm seeing you after a long time. How are you?

Mr. Khanna: I'm fine but there are some health problem in this age, well here is Muskan's gift. Where is she?

Sandeep: She is over there. Hello Mr. Harish, how are you? Please come and be seated, have some drinks. (To a child) well, you must be Pushkar, Muskan's class friend, 'go, she is over there.'

Ritu: Welcome Mrs. Jain. How are you!

Mrs. Jain: I'm fine Thank you.

Ritu: You seldom visit us now and I know even today it is because you had to accompany Tanya, (smiles).

And how are you Tanya baby? Go meet your friend Khushi and don't forget to wish her elder sister.

Mrs. Jain: you know Ritu. We <u>have</u> shifted to a far off place. That is why I don't visit you so often. Please accept Muskan's gift.

Ritu: Thank you, about the distance problem it is alright. I hope Mr. Jain is fine. Please be seated. We shall soon start games for children. Have something to drink.

(Sandeep is taking care of elderly people and some his friends. Ritu is organizing games for children.)

Ritu: Well children! There are folded slips in this basket. Come, pick them up and read what is written there. Each child will do what he/she is told. (Children pick up slips, open them and try to do what is written in them. Some have to dance, others tell jokes, sing act, laugh, weep etc. There is a lot of laughter and all enjoy.

Ritu: Now you can have some drinks and snacks to energize yourself for musical chairs and passing the pillow games.

(Children are busy in playing games. There is a lot of laughter and fun. There are quarrels and also even fisting.

Ritu expertly handles all such situations. In the meantime, the birthday cake arrives. All the guests gather around the cake. After lighting the candles, Muskan blows them out.)

All: Happy Birthday, Muskan.

                      (Muskan thanks them all, the cake is cut and pieces are distributed <u>to all the</u> children who <u>got busy</u> with more games.)

A lady guest: (to another) Ritu is so clever with children's games see how well she is managing the entire affair she sure has a way with children and they also like her.

Another one: Yes the children are having a <u>whale of time,</u> now they will always look forward to coming to Ritu's place. She <u>has</u> been organising such events <u>for</u> long. You see her daughter Khushi how cute she is!

Lady Guest: Yes but Muskan is <u>also</u> no less. You know she is a classmate of my son Vivek.

                      (After some time party gets over. Children receive their gifts from Ritu and Sandeep. Muskan and Khushi see off their friends. The elderly ones are given a warm good bye by the host couple.)

CHAPTER 7

A DINNER PARTY OF BUSINESS ASSOCIATES

Dinner parties are formal and they are also an exemplary example of social etiquette and balanced good behaviour and friendly camaraderie.

Mr. and Mrs. Sharma are standing at the gate and receiving guest.

Mr. Sandeep: Welcome Mr. Kashyap. I'm so glad that you have come. Welcome Mrs. Kashyap. Where are the kids?

Mrs. Kashyap: They have gone to their granny's house. You know these are holidays.

Ms. Ritu: Of course. Welcome Shivani! How are you?

Ms. Shivani: I'm fine Thank you. Congratulations your husband has got a new contract.

Ms. Ritu: Thanks. Where is your husband?

Ms Shivani: Don't worry; he'll be coming in a while.

(Soon the place is crowded and people start eating and talking.)

(Mr. Sandeep is keeping an eye over the place; he is also talking to the guests.)

Mr. Sandeep: (at the water counter) Why so few glasses, arrange for more. Is there enough mineral water?

Man: Yes, sir. More glasses have arrived and water is being filled in them.

Mr. Sandeep: (to a waiter) naan supply seems to be short, what's the matter? Call Mr. Malhotra.

Mr. Malhotra: Don't worry sir, we are working quickly. Dishes were tasted by Mrs. Sharma a short while ago. She has Ok'd them.

Mr. Sandeep: Good. Hello Vipul how are you? How is the food?

Vipul: Fine, everything is fine. I'm glad you got the contract. The race was tough. Do you know how many companies were in the <u>fray</u>?

Mr. Sandeep: I have some idea when our firm was shortlisted. I couldn't believe my eyes. Even now seems almost like a dream. Anyway how are things with you?

Vipul: (smiles) well I'm pulling on and waiting for a break.

Mr. Sandeep: Don't wait, attack.

(Sees a friend and business associate)

Please excuse, I'll be back in a short while. Hello Rishi, Namaste Bhabhiji, I can't believe you have <u>come</u> all the way from Singapore to attend the party.

Mr. Rishi:	(laughs) you're right. I had some work to attend to in Delhi. So I thought I'll <u>kill two birds with a stone.</u> (It is an idiom meaning to accomplish two tasks at one attempt.)
Mr. Sandeep:	We worked together last time. It was fine. What happened to the collaboration with that Architect firm in U.S.A.?
Mr. Rishi:	I'm working on it; I have strongly recommended your firm's name to them. Something will soon happen.
Mr. Sandeep:	Thanks. This Jaipur airport project is rather too much for me. But all the same, it has clicked. Rishi, do you see that gentleman near that table over there? Come let me introduce you. This man is <u>a winner hands down.</u>
	(It is an idiom meaning to accomplish two tasks at one attempt.)
Mr. Sandeep:	(to gentleman) Good evening Mr. Narayana. You have really done me great honour attending this humble party. Meet my friend and business associate Mr. Rishi, he is based in Singapore.
Rishi:	(shaking hands) Glad to meet you sir.
Mr. Narayana:	My pleasure. So you have done it Sandeep, I'm glad.
Mr. Sandeep:	Actually sir, had it not been for you, I would.......
Mr. Narayana:	Please! I only gave the matter a little push. Otherwise it was your hard work. Drop in at my office tomorrow. We may work out something new together.
Mr. Sandeep:	Sure sir that will be an honour. Please have food.
Mr. Narayana:	(smiles) Sure, that's what I have come here for.

An idioms meaning: A winner in all situations

Mr. Sandeep:	(to his partner) Hey Vineet, how are you? Have you eaten?
Mr. Vineet:	Yes I have yesterday. I checked the plan of the building, it seems alright. The owner Mr. Gupta is complaining in vain.
Mr. Sandeep:	I'll talk to him. Have you checked the central A.C. system, height of window, light arrangement, the cable and air ducts etc.
Mr. Vineet:	Yes, but nothing seems to please Mr. Gupta, we are professionals but he thinks himself above everybody.
Mr. Sandeep:	Oh! Chill out, I'll talk to him. (To a bunch of guests) How is everything? Please enjoy yourself. How is the food?
People around:	Very nice (all compliment Mr. Sandeep)

(The party draws to a close. Mr. and Mrs. Sandeep with everyone a hearty good bye and good night)

Sandeep:	(to an old gentleman) Bye Mr. Khurana.

(Calm down)

Shall I see you to your car? Where is your driver?

Mr. Khurana:	He is coming all the same. Thanks for your concern. It was a nice party.
Sandeep:	Thanks Mr. Khurana and bye, take care.

CHAPTER 8

A VISIT TO AGRA

Visiting tourist location needs us to be equipped with good communication skills to find our way around and interact fruitfully

(Sharma's of Delhi decide to visit Fatehpur Sikri and Taj Mahal by car. The occupants of the car are Sandeep Sharma his wife Ritu their two daughters Muskan and Khushi aged 11 and 5 and the parents of Sandeep. They are on their way to Agra)

Papa:	How much time do you think Sandeep, will it take for us to reach Agra?
Sandeep:	I guess five hours. It we take Taj Express Highway we'll make it sooner.
Papa:	I don't think it's open to public yet. Roll down the window. It's better if we ask for our way to Agra. (To a person standing by) could you please tell us which way is it Agra?
Person:	Go straight and then left. There is a Masjid also. Thank you. (They follow the route)
Ritu:	There is the Masjid. No need to ask now. The way to Agra is clearly written over there. The fellow was right.
Children:	We want our toffees and chewing gums.
Ritu:	No way, first eat some fruits and then take juice. After that we'll see. (All eat snacks and fruits)
Sandeep:	We are nearing Agra, must ask some person for way to Fatehpur. Hello! Could you tell us the road to Fatehpur Sikri?
Man:	Turn right and you'll find a signboard indicating the way. Actually it is a straight road from there.
Sandeep:	Thank you.

(As they near Fatehpur some people try to stop the car.)

Sandeep:	Yes?
One person:	You should park the car here. The parking fee is only hundred rupees.
Ritu:	Drive on Sandeep, these guys don't seem alright to me.
Sandeep:	(driving) But I see no vehicle here. All are going on foot.
Papa:	Just keep driving.

(As they reach Fatehpur a person beckons them)

A person:	You can park here. Buy from here a chuddar and flower for the Dargah.
Ritu:	How much for the chuddar?
The person:	Only 200 Rupees.

Ritu:	Make it half we shall buy otherwise there are others also.
The person:	Ok madam. Here is the chuddar and flowers. Please pay some money for the flowers.

Sandeep; Here is the Buland Darwaza. These are high stairs. Come give me your hand mummy. Papa is already ascending the stairs.

Khushi:	(at the gate) What are those things on the ceiling grandpa?
Grandpa:	They are hives of honeybees. You must have read or heard about them. They are clever to make their hives so high; otherwise people will just break them and take away the honey. (Many people on the floor are selling necklaces and bangles along with other fancy items children are fascinated.)

Ritu; don't be so excited, we shall buy something after we have visited the Dargah. Shall we hire a guide Sandeep?

Sandeep:	By all means. The place fascinates me. (They hire a guide)
Guide:	Sir this building is called Fatehpur Sikri is the place around here. Do you see those plains below? Babar fought a war with the local kings. He defeated them and started to build their structure as a mark his victory. Later it was completed by other kings......
Sandeep:	(on their way back to a person as they way the city) could you please tell in the way of Taj?
The person:	Turn left, after about a kilometer ask for the place from where the battery train leaves for Taj.
Sandeep:	Thanks.
Ritu:	I think I saw the place on our way to Fatehpur Sikri. There is a restaurant also. We'll take our lunch there.

(In the restaurant)

Sandeep:	(to the waiter) please bring the menu and give us water.
Waiter:	Yes sir.
Ritu:	(reads the menu card) Bring us two dals, two vegetables, shahi paneer and raita. Also bring ten chapattis. At the end bring a large limca bottle.
Sandeep:	(after the lunch) Please bring our bill. Also tell us from where to buy tickets for train to Taj.
Waiter:	Just outside sir.
Ritu:	(at the ticket window) Four tickets please and two for children. Khushi and Muskan you go and fill your water bottle from that tap.

(During the train ride)

Papa:	What a smokeless and noiseless cute little train.
Driver:	Now this is the only means to reach Taj because earlier The Taj had begun to <u>lose</u> its shine because of the petrol and diesel smoke.
Papa:	A sensible thing to do.

(Train stops and they are frisked at the by policeman)

Policeman:	to grandpa, these chocolates etc, Can't take them inside.
Grandpa:	Why? These are for children quite harmless.
Policeman:	Rules sir. We have to follow them. Please go out and deposit them with some shopkeeper.
Grandpa:	It is ridiculous. (He goes out) (Before entering Taj they all wear plastic covering over their shoes)

A Japanese tourist to Sandeep: Could you please tell me something about the beautiful building.

Sandeep:	Sure, you may hire a guide as well.
Tourist:	Yes but I find it difficult to follow them.
Sandeep:	(to the family) meet me down stairs in half an hour.
Sandeep:	Well, Emperor Shah Jahan built this great monument in memory of beloved queen Mumtaj. It took 22 years and 22000 people to build it. Experts and rare pieces of stone were brought from Iran and other countries. You see how perfectly circular is the dome and symmetrical the four minarets. The workers.......

(The family unites downstairs and they come out.)

Khushi:	Dada, please bring our chocolates and toffees.
Grandpa:	Sorry child! I almost forgot them. Go towards the train, I'm going to bring them.
Khushi:	(to lady in the train) Aunty please take some other seat. We want to enjoy the ride sitting at the rear end, come Muskan didi.
Lady:	(smiles) Of course child. It's all yours. I'll take some other seat. (On their way back to Delhi the Sharma's pass the Red Fort)
Muskan:	Papa you promised me a visit to the Red Fort also. Let's go there.
Sandeep:	Sorry Muskan. We are all tired. Besides it's a very big building and we have to reach Delhi by night all.

Muskan; Oh, papa! At least show me the place where Shahjahan was kept prisoner by his son and from where he could his believe Taj Mahal in a small piece of glass.

Sandeep:	That is how the story goes but not this time Muskan. It will be the first place to see when we visit Agra next.

(At night on the highway)

Ritu:	Something wrong with the car Sandeep. It's slowing down. (The car stops) Oh god! What shall we do now? There is no mechanic here and it is so dark. Why didn't you check the tyre at the last dhaba we stopped?
Sandeep:	I should have. Anyway all of you stay in the car. Don't open the door it is a busy highway. (He gets down and checks the tyres). Nothing to worry we have got a <u>flat tyre.</u> I'll fix it. Papa come out carefully, help me. (They take out the jack and another tyre from the dickey and fix the new wheel).
Papa:	(On back) we were lucky. It was only a damaged tyre and not some trouble in the engine. Thank god! (Flat means punctured tyre.)

CHAPTER 9

REPORTING THE LOSS OF A.T.M CARD IN BANK

The need to maintain equanimity in the times of adversity is a paramount need and necessity for positive social interaction and satisfactory outcome.

Customer: (to the clerk) I have lost my A.T.M card.

Clerk: Please go to that counter and talk to Mr. Gupta.

Customer: (to Mr. Gupta) Sir. I have lost my A.T.M card please tell me the procedure of how to get a new one.

Mr. Gupta: Ok. Do you have the balance slip from the A.T.M machine?

Customer: Yes sir there it is.

Mr. Gupta: Very well, you see this phone number at the bottom. Instruct the person at this phone number to block your A.T.M card so that no other person can use it. Tell him your account number.

Customer: After that, Sir?

Mr. Gupta: He'll give you a number note it down carefully. Then write an application to the manager of the bank. In the application quote that code number along with the request to issue you a new A.T.M card.

Customer: How much time will it take to get me a new card?

Mr. Gupta: Ten or fifteen days after you have submitting the application to us. After that you'll receive a letter from the bank. Bring it here. (After ten days the customer A.K Gupta gets a letter from the bank.)

Mr. Jain: (to Mr. Gupta) there is the letter sir.

Mr. Gupta: Your driving license or your election id card. The bank wants to make sure that the card goes to the right person. Have you brought your bank passbook?

Mr. Jain: Yes sir.

Mr. Gupta: Very well show all those documents to Mr. Sharma.

(Mr. Jain shows the paper to Mr. Sharma)

Mr. Sharma: All right Mr. Jain a moment please. (Takes and a register and finds his name). Please sign against your name. (Mr. Gupta does so.) Here is your envelope. Open it carefully preferable at home in privacy because it contains your ATM card as well as the ATM pin number. None other than you must know that number. The fee of the new card is Rs. 200. The amount will be deducted from your account. Open the envelope carefully.

Mr. Jain: Thank you Mr. Sharma.

Mr. Sharma: It is alright.

CHAPTER 10

LODGING AN FIR AT THE POLICE STATION

The need to rope in the law where it is necessary and to do it with the best possible skills in communication and ensuring that at no point of time we hurt or anger the sentiments of law.

A man:	(to another outside the police station) Where to go for lodging an FIR?
Another man:	What have you lost?
First man:	My driving license.
Second man:	Where?
First man:	I don't remember, may be somewhere at the bus stand.
Second man:	Don't mention that to the policeman at the duty. Tell him you left it at home. That will make things easy.
First man:	Thank you.
Second man:	That's alright. You see that counter over there? There are three or four policeman sitting there. Go talk to anyone of them.
First man:	(to a policeman Sitting behind the table) Sir, I want to lodge a report. I have lost my Driving license.
Policeman:	Your name please? And where do you live?
Man:	My name is Rajiv Dua and I live in Geeta colony.
Policeman:	When and where did you lose it?
Mr. Dua:	At home, Sir, only a few days ago.
Policeman:	Well write down an application mentioning all the details your name, Father's name, addresses, when and where you lost it etc. Address it to the SHO.

(Mr. Dua asks for a paper and writes down an application mentioning necessary details and hands it over to the policeman.

Policeman:	(after reading it) have you got a zerox copy of the lost license.
Mr. Dua:	No, sir.
Policeman:	Do so in further. It makes things easy.
Mr. Dua:	Yes sir. When shall I get the report?
Policeman:	The report will be prepared at the computer or you can say it will be a computerized report. Wait for an hour or you can come tomorrow.
Mr. Dua:	Thanks sir. I'll prefer to wait.

A FAMILY AT BREAKFAST

A family get together is the most interactive place in a day. It's the time when we interact with all the members of the family and share our day to day life proceedings with opinions and advice galore.

Mother:	Good morning Tina, good morning Rahul isn't it time you got up?
Children:	Morning mom.
Mother:	Please don't leave your bed unmade. It's a bad habit. Smoothen the bed sheet put the pillows right and properly fold the covering sheets. Kindly attend to your daily morning routine after that.
Tina:	Where is my toothpaste?
Rahul:	And where is my towel?
Mother:	Learn to take care of your things. You're grown up children now. Rahul look into your drawer. Your towel may be there and Tina you can take toothpaste from my bedroom. Are your shoes polished Rahul?
Rahul:	Oh! I forgot mummy. I'll just polish them before taking bath.
Mother:	Ok, after taking bath arrange your school bags and come for breakfast.

(Mother lays the breakfast table)

Tina:	What is there in breakfast mom?
Mother:	Omelet and two glassful of milk for you two.
Father:	(enters in a hurry) sorry dear, can I have my breakfast too. Oh! I forgot to tell you that I have a meeting at sharp 9'o' clock.
Mother:	You should have told me. I'm attending to children. They shouldn't be late for school. Please help yourself to the fridge, take out the juice and here are a couple of sandwiches.
Tina:	Here is your coffee mom. I would love to serve you but it is already our school time.
Mother:	It's alright dear, thanks. I appreciate your sentiments.

Chapter 12

AN INTERVIEW SCENE

A good conversation demands a certain strength — the strength to feel comfortable with someone else; the strength to remain in and of oneself even while being so intent on another; the strength to enter strange, new realms without getting lost. It demands that peculiar posture of poise, leaning neither too far in nor too far back but standing strong while always ready for what may come next.

Candidate: (to clerk) my name is R.K Gupta. I have been called here for interview.

Clerk: (checks in the list) Yes, your name is there. Please sit down. I'll call you as soon as your turn comes.

R.K Gupta: Thanks.

Clerk: (after sometime) You can go in now Mr. Gupta.

R.K Gupta: (enters after knocking) Good morning gentleman.

One member of the interview board: Good morning please have a seat. Your name is R.K Gupta?

R.K Gupta: Yes sir, my name is R.K Gupta. Thank you very much for calling me to interview.

Second member: That's alright, what is your educational qualifications?

R.K Gupta: Sir I am M.A, B.ed.

Third member: Where did you study?

R.K Gupta: Sir, I did my graduation and post graduation in English from K.M college, Delhi university. I did my B.ed from the same university, central institute of education.

Fourth member: Good, what are you technical subjects?

R.K Gupta: English and Political science in B.A.

Third member: Why did you choose this profession?

R.K Gupta: Sir I think that teaching is a very noble profession. Here you have a great opportunity of shaping the career and character of youngsters who are going to be builder of our nation.

Second member: What are your hobbies?

R.K Gupta: Reading, writing, travelling and teaching of course. I want to make it my career as well.

First member: Thanks, Mr. Gupta. You can go now we'll let you know about the result.

INTRODUCTION TO A FAMILY

A family get together is the most interactive place in a day. It's the time when we interact with all the members of the family and share our day to day life proceedings with opinions and advice galore.

House lady:	(open the door after hearing the bell) Yes?
Stranger:	You're Mamta aunty, aren't you?
Mrs. Kaushik:	Yes I am. Who are you?
Stranger:	I'm Deepak. You know Lata aunty in Agra; I'm her brother-in-law's son.
Mrs. Kaushik:	Oh! You're Rajeev's son, come in please.
Deepak:	Thanks aunty.
Mrs. Kaushik:	How is everybody in Agra?
Deepak:	All are fine.
Mrs. Kaushik:	(leading him to breakfast table) You are at the right time. All the family is here. Listen, everybody this boy is in my distant relation. You children can consider him your cousin. Deepak kindly introduce yourself.
Deepak:	Good morning everybody. (All say,' good morning. He sits at the table) my name is Deepak Arya. I live in Agra near Radha swami complex. My father Anil Kumar Arya is a doctor having his own practise. My mother is a house lady. I have a sister and a brother both are studying in school. I have passed my 12th grade and have appeared in joint entrance examination for MBBS. Aunty here is some petha and namkeen my mother has sent for you. I convey her best wishes to all of you.
Mr. Kaushik:	Thanks to your mom Deepak. Please sit down and enjoy the breakfast with us. I'll introduce the member of our family to you.
Mr. Kaushik's son:	Brother Deepak. I hope you will be staying with us for some time. We are all so eager to hear about Taj Mahal, Red Fort and Fatehpur Sikri Agra is a great historical city. It has always fascinated me.
Deepak:	Sure, I hope all of us will spend a lot of happy time together.

CHAPTER 14

A DIALOGUE BETWEEN FATHER AND DAUGHTER

A conversation between father and his daughter invariably discusses future prospects advice and exchange of views and opinions.

Papa:	(to his daughter) Reena, yesterday you again scolded your brother Ritika and that too very harshly.
Reena:	What shall I do papa? He does so many stupid things that I just can't stand them.
Papa:	Look Reena he is a very gentle boy and I would say rather a good one. Harsh rebukes will only produce negative results. I have told you so many times to check your anger but you don't listen to me. You'll agree with me that anger is a negative emotion.
Reena:	(after a pause) Yes, papa. There you are right. But again he never does things in time. He'll start doing his homework at either lunch or dinner time. Mom will keep calling him and he won't listen. Yesterday I had a quarrel with him right over this point.
Papa:	I agree. But have you notice that he has begun to talk back. That's not a good sign. Either you deal with him gently or let your mother handle him.
Reena:	If I complain to mom. Then also he gets upset. Have you seen papa how shabby his room is? All his clothes, books etc, are lying helter skelter.
Papa:	Ok, I'll talk to him but stop picking quarrels with him. The whole house gets disturbs. Nobody is fault free, at least he doesn't criticize you or does he?
Reena:	No, papa but then I'm his elder sister.
Papa:	Right, so maintain that dignity. Talk to him soberly. That will produce good results.
Reena:	Ok papa, I'll try my best.

A DIALOGUE BETWEEN MOTHER AND SON

A conversation between mother and her son invariably discusses future prospects advice and exchange of views and opinions.

Mother: (to son) you're late Sonu. It is 3'o' clock now, your exam must have been over by 1'o' clock.

Sonu: Oh! Mom I begun to play in the school!

Mother: You should have told me.

Sonu: How mom? Some students were playing badminton and they invited me. <u>I couldn't help it</u>, you know our PTI sir is very good. He says that after the exam, students should relax a bit. He gives us net badminton rackets and......

Mother: Ok, ok tell me about your exam.

Sonu: It went well. I knew most of the answers.

Mother: That's good. In future don't overstay in school. How are your studies going?
I had to do it.

Sonu: All right. Most of our teachers good, except that of Sanskrit.

Mother: What's the matter?

Sonu: Many times he doesn't take class. He is busy with some school work. You know Sanskrit so well, mom. Why don't you help me cover the topic?

Mom: I'll gladly do that. How is you friend circle?

Sonu: They are all good boys except Nigam. He criticizes me and talks ill of me behind my back. Besides, he is the monitor of the class and bit of a bully.

Mom: I'll talk to your class teacher and I think I know his mother. I'll talk to her also. Sonu choose you friends wisely, a person is knows by the company he keeps. Besides bad friends, inculcate bad habits and yours is a very impressionable age.

Sonu: I'll be careful mom.

Mom: Good also don't avoid the glass of milk at your breakfast table. I know you like tea, but that is ruled out.

Sonu: All right mom but can I drink tea on Sundays.

Mom: Ok, also don't keep late hours. You usually sleep late. I hope you aren't into reading novels.

Sonu: No mom. But sometimes I do read Hardy boys novel, they are good.

Mom: No harm, but don't make it a habit and do not exceed the time limit of two hours' play in the evening stick strictly to the time table, I have made for you.

Sonu: Ok mom I'll do that.

CONVERSATION BETWEEN HUSBAND AND WIFE

This kind of conversation invariably leads to arguments or discussion regarding household matters

Husband: Good morning dear.

Wife: Good morning. Here is your favorite breakfast a hamburger, coffee and a glass of pomegranate juice.

Husband: Fine, thank you. You seem to have woken up rather early.

Wife: Yes I have to prepare some special lunch for children. Their class is going for picnic.

Husband; I see. (Pause) How are their studies going?

Wife; Fine Sanjay has some problem in maths while Ajay is lagging behind in science.

Husband: So what is to be done?

Wife: I am trying to find a tutor who can teach the boys both maths and science; it's not much of a problem I'll see to it. Sometimes you should also talk to them about their problems, their teacher, friends and hobbies etc.

Husband: I'll do that. How about home budget? We had decided to clear our home loan before time.

Wife: I think I can manage home with lesser amount. I have stopped going to kitty parties. I find them boring. I'll be able to give more time to house and children. That will save money. I think I can do without maid, she has grown very irregular.

Husband: Well if you can manage and I know you will. You do have a knack for it. But please don't tire yourself, too much work can tax mind and body. I want you to be relaxed and happy. May be I can work overtime.

Wife: Please don't, you're already overburdened in office and come late. I have found a new provisional store at very moderate rates. I'll start shopping there. For the coming six months, we need nothing extra besides our regular usual budget. So we can clear our loans. I hope you're satisfied with the food and the way our home is being run.

Husband: (smiles) Oh! You are excellent darling to the extent of the being faultless. I began to love you more.

Wife: (blushes) I must go and wake up the children. Could you come rather early from office today?

Husband: I can manage. Any event?

Wife:	No we will talk to our children and chalk further schemes of saving money. I'm running out of vegetables and fruits. See if you can bring something.
Husband:	I'll surely do that. After all you seldom ask me to do such things shall I bring you your favourite *kanji burin* and a *gajara* full of fragrant flowers. You look so beautiful when you wear it.
Wife:	(smiles) you can't help being romantic. But no complaints. Do as you wish. It's time you were leaving for office and I am going to wake up children. Bye dear.
Husband:	Bye, see you in the evening.

Chapter 12

CONVERSATION BETWEEN HUSBAND AND WIFE WITH THEIR CHILDREN

Also known as the house parliament, this type of conversation is about future plans be it holiday or outing or any kind of family gathering or function.

Father: Well Sumit, what are your plans for future?

Sumit: After my 12th I plan to do BCA and find a job in an MNC.

Mother: But sometime back Sumit you told me you were planning to get into Air Force.

Sumit: Yes, but I'm undecided.

Sister: Papa Sumit's weight can be a problem in physical tests in Air Force.

Father: You're right. Can you reduce Sumit?

Sumit: I can but then it has to be a life long effort, more over since I began to do computers in school. I have developed a fascination for them.

Father; Well then you go for computers. Drop the Air Force idea.

Mother: What about you Nidhi?

Nidhi: I have no head for computers. I'm fond of English language and for that matter any other language like Spanish, French. You know mom they are teaching us French in school.

Father: That's good. But what career do you intend to take up?

Sumit: Dad I think she should graduate in English honors and then plan ahead.

Nidhi: Yes it can be but I would rather learn a couple of languages and become an interpreter. There are lots of vacancies in private and public sectors with handsome salaries and honourable posts.

Mother: Not a bad idea. I think you should go for it Nidhi.

Father: Yes everyone to him or her taste.

ASKING FOR BUS ROUTE AT CHANDNI CHOWK

When making new friends, there are usually three parts to the conversation you will have with your new friend. The first is the greeting. In this part, you and your new friend will greet each other and tell each other your names. The second part is the conversation. Sometimes the conversation is small talk and sometimes the conversation is about important matters, the third part of the conversation is the leave-taking. In this part, you tell your new friend that you are happy to meet him and that you must end the conversation.

A person:	(to a passer- by) Excuse me, could you please tell me how to reach Nehru Place.
Passer by:	Well, you can catch the metro from here (pointing to the metro station) but you'll have to change at Rajiv Chowk.
The person:	Yes, do you see the Red Fort from here? Go straight cross the road. You'll find many bus stands there. You can further enquire from there.
The person:	Thank you (at Red Fort bus stand from another person) from where can I get bus for Nehru Place?
Other person:	You can get the bus from that third stand from here.
The person:	Thanks. (From the conductor) will this bus go to Nehru Place?
Conductor:	No but you can board bus number 763 from here. You can get into a blue line or a red line.
The person:	What's the difference?
A person:	(standing nearby) the red bus will charge you double the fare, it's air conditioned. The blue one has normal rates. Both are comfortable buses. Look! Here comes the blue line get into it it'll go to Nehru place.
The person:	(boarding the bus) Thanks a lot. (Inside the bus to the conductor)

Please give me a ticket for Nehru Place and tell me when we reach there. I am new here.

Conductor:	(giving the ticket) Sit over there you. I'll tell when we reach Nehru Place.

A HOSPITAL SCENARIO

This place could be grim and hold unhappy prospects so when you do ask a question that can be answered in a single word, instead of just supplying your own information in response, ask a follow-up question.

Visitor:	(to the receptionist) could you please tell me where Mr. H.K. Sareen is admitted.
Receptionist:	Please tell the full name and the date when the patient was admitted.
Visitor:	Well the name Harish Kumar Sareen and he was admitted yesterday.
Receptionist:	(after checking in computer) it is ward no -4, room no 416.
Visitor:	How do I find it?
Receptionist:	Go straight and enter the door marked 'Orthopedics.' Ask any ward boy there and he will guide you.
Visitor:	Thanks. (Inside from any employee) Could you please guide me to ward no. 4, room number416?
Employee:	Turn to your left and then straight.
Visitor:	Thanks.
Visitor:	(inside the room) Good morning aunty. How is uncle now? What happened?
Aunt:	Well Govind your uncle's bike slipped and he fracture his leg.
Govind:	Uncle seems to be sleeping. I hope it is nothing serious.
Aunt:	No by God's grace it is not he has been given sedatives. But he will be kept here for a few days.
Govind:	(to doctor who has just entered) Good morning doctor. I'm the patient's nephew. I hope nothing is serious.
Doctor:	Don't worry. It is a simple fracture; we have set the bone and plastered his leg. Fortunately he was admitted here very quickly after the accident.
Govind:	When could he leave, sir?
Doctor:	In a few days, I hope. Since he has hurt his back also, we are keeping him under observation for a few days.
Govind:	Thank you sir. Aunty you can rest for a while I'm here.
Aunty:	Oh! It is alright. Can you bring these medicines from downstairs? Here is the money.
Govind:	Sure, aunty, no problem.

IN CONSULTATION WITH A DOCTOR

This type of conversation needs to brief, to the point. One has to tell his physical and mental ailments in details and also the symptoms of the affected disease to the doctor on a phone call.

Patient: I have not been feeling well for the last few days.

Doctor: Tell me about it:

Patient: (cough) you see doctor there is this cough, also I'm feeling cold all the time although it is no season for cold.

Doctor: (checks his BP and temperature) Your BP is alright but you are running a mild temperature. Anywhere pain in the body.

Patient: Not pain at any exact place but all the time I seem run down and exhausted. I'm restless even in bed.

Doctor: For how many days it has been like that?

Patient: Well two, three days.

Doctor: Take out your tongue and let me see your throat. (Checks) well it seems to me a mild sort of throat infection. Is there any other thing that you would like to tell me?

Patient: As I told you, I feel restless, exhausted and cough at times – a sort of burning sensation in throat which might have caused this throat infection. I'm very careful about not eating or drinking out.

Doctor: You can never say. Sometimes you can even inhale germs sometimes the throats get irritated by spices or very cold drinks. Here take these tablets and syrup three times a day and come tomorrow.

Patient: I hope it is nothing serious.

Doctor: Oh no! It's just an ordinary infection. Avoid chilies, sour things and cold water. You'll be alright within a few days.

Patient: Thanks doctor.

TELEPHONIC TALK WITH DOCTOR ABOUT SEVERE STOMACH PAIN

The conversation needs to be clear concise and to the point, namely questions and answers about medicines, food, etc.

Patient: Hello doctor, I'm having severe stomach ache. Can you do something about it?

Doctor: From where are you speaking?

Patient: Sector 44 R, K Puram. It is not very far from your clinic but I can't come. Please tell me some medicine so that the pain goes away.

Doctor: It is very difficult to say something on phone without proper check up. What is your name and age?

Patient: My name is Rajesh and I am 35. Please doctor do tell me some treatment on phone as soon as the pain lessens, I'll come to your clinic.

Doctor: Ok what sort of pain you have, are you having loose motions or is it constipation?

Patient: None, my stomach feels heavy like a stone and the pain comes and goes.

Doctor: Well, don't drink or eat anything. Is there a chemist nearby?

Patient: Yes I can manage to walk a little.

Doctor: Ok buy a medicine 'Spasmindon! It is liquid; take a few drop of it with warm water. That will reduce the pain, after that come for a check up.

Patient: If the pain stops even then I have to come?

Doctor: Yes, it might be severe stomach infection which will have to be treated with medicines. It might take you 3-4 days to get alright.

Patient: I'll do that. Thanks doctor.

A VISIT TO FRIEND'S SICK MOTHER

This place could be grim and hold unhappy prospects, so when you do ask a question that can be answered in a single word, instead of just supplying your own information in response, ask a follow-up question.

Vipul:	How is your mother these days, Ketan, last time you told me she had some sort of pain in joints.
Ketan:	Well she has that pain, I showed her to an orthopedic and he diagnosed it Ostoarthritis.
Vipul:	Is it something serious?
Ketan:	Yes and no. It you attend a physiotherapy clinic and then do the prescribed exercise at home it can be checked, but it is not curable.
Vipul:	That is not good news. Are you going home? I would like to accompany you.
Ketan:	you're welcome.

(After reaching home)

Vipul:	How are you feeling aunty? I heard from Ketan that you were not well.
Ketan's mother:	(smiles) it is not much of a bother. Most of the people in old age or even middle age get it.
Vipul:	What does the doctor say; Ketan tells me there is no cure for it.
Mother:	Yes, but with exercises it can be checked.
Vipul:	How are you feeling now? Is there much pain?
Mother:	There is no pain when I'm sitting or lying but walking has become an effort.
Vipul:	Any medicines that the doctor has prescribed.
Mother:	Yes, I'm taking them regularly and the pain is much less.
Vipul:	That is good. Show me your walk aunty.
Aunty:	(gets up with an effort there is a slight limp) you see son, I can walk but with an effort.
Vipul:	Oh! Aunty, it seems nothing serious I'm sure you'll be alright with regular medication and exercises. I know a renowned Vaidya I'll talk to him about you.
Aunty:	God bless you my son and thanks for coming.

PURCHASES FROM GENERAL MERCHANT

A conversation demands great generosity. On the one hand, it demands the generosity of listening. And perhaps not just of listening but of assuming that the other person is saying something of value, something worth listening to.

(Customer Darshan Singh talks to general merchant Kishan lal)

Darshan:	How are you Kishan?
Kishan:	I'm alright what shall I give you.
Darshan:	(reading from a list) tamarind worth ten rupees.
Kishan:	It is in a pack of 20 rupees. We don't sell loose.
Darshan:	Ok but you do sell loose ghee, give me 250 gms. How much for it?
Kishan:	65 rupees.
Darshan:	Three bars of surf excel soap, ½ kg dal each of *rajma, arhar, urad, chana*, ½ kg of tata tea. By the way any scheme over it?
Kishan:	No not on tata tea but on other brands there is.
Darshan:	No let it be tata. How much in this *kasoori methi* pack?
Kishan:	Only ten rupees.
Darshan:	Ok how about that *garam masala* pack, it is MDH isn't it.
Kishan:	Ten rupees only.
Darshan:	Ok give ½ kg Surf washing powder, these spices 100 gms. Each (gives him a list), one big brown bread, 200 gms of butter and that mango pickle jar how much for it?
Kishan:	Only eighty rupees for ½ kg.
Darshan:	That is quite fair; give me that pack of papads and that chana masala packet, Half kg of white grams also
Kishan:	Anything else?
Darshan:	Yes one ten rupees limca bottle.
Kishan:	We no longer keep small bottles. Only 1 ltr bottle worth rupees 60.
Darshan:	Ok put all these items in this bag and the bill please.
Kishan:	There it is, only 650 rupees.

A DISCUSSION AMONG FRIENDS

Small talk is used at parties, when meeting people, etc. to be kind and get along with others at the events. Hopefully, small talk leads to more interesting conversations. However, the ability to small talk and use appropriate phrases can help get the conversation flowing.

Rakesh:	We have met at the right place. This cross river mall is one of the best I have known.
Sushant:	You're right. Shall we make some purchases?
Rajan:	What an array of shirts and trousers and what classy crowd here!
Shrikant:	Alas! We can only see them, buying is a dream. Popular brands will start anywhere from 2 to 3 thousand.
Rajan:	Let's go to Laxmi nagar V3S cinema. We can buy something at a Nirman Vihar outlet as well as watch a movie.
Rajan:	(at V3S mall) Sushant you go in and buy for 4 p.m. movie show tickets, by that time, we'll finish shopping and eating. There is a McDonald outlet very near in Preet vihar.
Shrikant:	(in the mall) How much is this shirt.
Salesman:	One thousand rupees.
Shrikant:	It's costly here. Rajan where is the place where we could buy something at a less price.
Rajan:	Right there across the street. You see there is 50% discount with luck we can find a popular brand shirt or jeans. But wait Sushant is coming. Have you got the tickets?
Sushant:	Yes where to now?

(They all move inside and make some purchases)

Shrikant:	This is a good place, nice stuff at almost half the price.
Sushant:	I'm hungry as well as thirsty. Let's go to the restaurant now.

(Inside McDonald)

Rajan:	The vegetable hamburger at Rs. 30 seems very good. Four hamburgers and four cokes, Ok? It's self help here, so I'm getting the stuff.

(All nod)

Shrikant:	see those foreigners, if we listen to them carefully, we can improve our accent and vocabulary a lot.
Rajan:	Sushant come here and carry these plates.

(After the restaurant and movie)

Sushant:	Shall we part ways or any other plans?
Shrikant:	What about Ansal Plaza, It is fantastic there sitting in the open on the full moon night.
Sushant:	Good idea. I would like to visit the Reebok shop there. They are offering huge discount sale.

PARENTS-TEACHER MEETING IN SCHOOL

React to what the teacher says to you as a parent in the spirit in which that comment was offered and continue with the flow of the conversation.

Sudha: (to teacher) Good morning ma'm. I'm Sudha Nidhi's mother, this is her father. She is in class 8th B. Please tell us how she is doing in her subjects.

Teacher: (turning the pages) she is Nidhi Aggarwal, isn't she? Well so far as her performance in tests is concerned, it is not very satisfactory.

Mr. Aggarwal: Please tell us about exam results and her over all Performance.

Teacher: On the whole she is good. Her attendance is regular, behaviour, discipline is good. But she is lagging behind in science and maths.

Sudha: What about other subjects?

Teacher: She is good. In the three class tests of 60 marks she got 50 in Sanskrit, 45 in English and 40 in Hindi.

Mr. Aggarwal: How is extra curricular activities.

Teacher: She is very good, especially in drama; she is good in sports also.

Sudha: Does she adjust well with her class mates?

Teacher: Oh yes, she is very friendly with almost all of them.

Mrs. & Mr. Aggarwal: Thanks ma'm and bye.

Chapter 26

CAREER COUNSELLING

This kind of conversation is different than a discussion. In career counselling, experts or counsellors talk and advise the students to opt for their choice of subjects and continue their higher education, and make a career for themselves.

Lokesh:	Good morning sir could you spare me a little time. I want to consult you about my career.
Counsellor:	Sure, What is your qualification and age?
Lokesh:	I'm eighteen sir, I have passed my 12th in Arts stream.
Counsellor:	Well any career in accountancy or medicine is ruled out. What is your percentage?
Lokesh:	Average 85% in all subjects.
Counsellor:	Good you can go in teaching line. You can do graduation with honors in your favorite subjects.
Lokesh:	No sir, I don't have any aptitude for that.
Counselor:	What about appearing in Defense services exams.
Lokesh:	No sir, I do not keep very good health, besides my eye sight is weak.
Counsellor:	Do you like computers?
Lokesh:	Yes sir I like computer operating.
Counsellor:	Well then you can do BCA from IGNOU. You can get admission in any university because your percentage is good. After BCA or MCA you can get a handsome job in any MNC. How is your drawing? Was it one of your subjects?
Lokesh:	I'm very good at drawing.
Counselor:	Good then you can go in architecture line also. Your expertise in computers will be of great help.
Lokesh:	That seems a good idea, sir. Where should I apply?
Counsellor:	There is a School of Architecture and Planning at ITO crossing. Go there with your certificates and testimonials. I hope the admission still open, fill up the application form for admission.
Lokesh:	Any other institute in Delhi.
Counsellor:	No, but you can go to Nasik if you don't get admission here. Nasik Architecture School has a very good reputation.
Lokesh:	Thank sir, I'll do as you advice.

FIRST DAY OF A STUDENT IN A COLLEGE

Small talk is used at parties, when meeting people, etc. to be kind and get along with others at the events. Hopefully, small talk leads to more interesting conversations. However, the ability to small talk and use appropriate phrases can help get the conversation flowing.

A student:	(nervously looks at the crowd and consciously approaches a boy standing apart) Hello!
Other students:	Hello, are you new here?
First student:	Yes my name is Mukesh.
Other student:	I am Akash.
Mukesh:	(shakes his hand) Glad to see you. What is your subject?
Akash:	B.Com, what is yours?
Mukesh:	English Honours. It is my first day here and I'm feeling very nervous, like a fish out of water.
Akash:	The same here, but nervousness is of no use, rather it may be to our disadvantage.
Mukesh:	Right, have you heard about ragging! Nervous new comes like us are sitting targets!
Akash:	Come let's go and sit in the garden out there.
(Both sit on a bench)	
Mukesh:	From which school did you pass your 12th?
Akash:	Anglo Sanskrit school in Daryaganj.
Mukesh:	I'm from SBV, R.K. Puram.
Akash:	I looked at the notice board but couldn't locate my class. Did you try?
Mukesh:	(laughs) Yes and I also failed. There is so much crowd here. Why not leave now and come tomorrow.
(A burly fellow approaching them)	
Fellow:	Are you guys new here?
Both:	(nervously standing up) Yes sir.
Fellow:	(laughs) I'm your senior we're parading the fresher's here come get up.
Both:	(very nervously) please let's go sir.
Fellow:	(again laughs) I was joking. Actually I have been deputed by the principal to check out if there is any ragging. Be at ease, I'm Sanjeev Mehta. 3rd year B.Com. (Shakes hands with them)
Mukesh:	Sir, I was looking for my class. I'm also a B.Com student. Could you help us, Akash is English honors.
Sanjeev:	Come with me. I'll help you.

BOY TALKING TO A GIRL IN COLLEGE

When making new friends, there are usually three parts to the conversation you will have with your new friend. The first is the *greeting*. In this part, you and your new friend will greet each other and tell each other your names. The second part is the *conversation*. Sometimes, the conversation is *small talk* and sometimes the conversation is about *important matters*, the third part of the conversation is the *leave-taking*. In this part, you tell your new friend that you are happy to meet him and that you must end the conversation.

A first year student: Excuse me; did Mr. Kohli take class yesterday?

Girl:	Do I know you?
Boy:	I am Kunal Kapoor. We study in the same class. Sorry for the botheration, I didn't come to college yesterday.
Girl:	Mr. Kohli took the class.
Kunal:	(after a pause) did you attend his class?
Girl:	Yes.
Kunal:	You must have taken notes if it is not much of trouble could I have a look at them. Mr. Kohli is my favorite lecture. I never miss his classes.
Girl:	He is my favorite too. Let me see where his notes are. By the way I'm Sanjana Garg.
Kunal:	Glad to meet you Sanjana.
Sanjana:	(opening a page in the notebook) Here you are.
Kunal:	Thanks, I'll give it back to you in a short while. If you don't mind, let's make a pact.
Sanjana:	What pact?
Kunal:	Whenever one of us misses Mr. Kohl's lecture. The other one will help him or her with notes.
Sanjana:	Agreed. It's time for class now, bye!
Kunal:	Bye!

A MAN IN A HOTEL

Small talk is used at parties, when meeting people, etc. to be kind and get along with others at the events. Hopefully, small talk leads to more interesting conversations. However, the ability to small talk and use appropriate phrases can help get the conversation flowing.

Man: (to hotel receptionist) Excuse me, is there a room booked in the name Roshan Taneja.

Receptionist: One moment, sir. (Checks) No sir, I'm sorry there is no such booking. May I know your name sir?

Man: I'm Roshan Taneja, I myself booked a room here.

Receptionist: Can you tell me the room number?

Mr. Taneja: No I don't have it.

Receptionist: That is it. Actually sir you didn't confirm the booking.

Mr. Taneja: I see. So what happens now? I want a room and it is urgent.

Receptionist: Let me see. What we can do for you.

Mr. Taneja: Please.

Receptionist: (after a while) Right now there is no room vacant sir, I'm sorry. But should you wait a while. One customer is about to check out. You want a single room isn't it? Please have a seat.

Mr. Taneja: It's alright I'll wait. (Waits)

Receptionist: Here you're Mr. Taneja. You're lucky. The customer has checked out. Yours room is no 203. Will you please fill up this form? This boy here will escort you to your room. He'll also carry your baggage. Have you an ID card?

Mr. Taneja: (filling the form) Here is my Id and thanks.

Receptionist: You're welcome.

CHAPTER 30

TALK WITH A PROPERTY DEALER FOR BUYING A HOUSE

You do ask a *question* that can be answered in a single word, instead of just supplying your own information in response, ask a *follow-up question*.

Customer : (to the property dealer) I want to buy a two room house.

Property dealer : you mean 2 BHK, Sir, i.e., two bedrooms, kitchen and a hall or drawing room.

Customer : Yes, that is it.

Dealer : Which floor and in what locality?

Customer: In Geeta Colony or say in a radius of one km, not farther than that. I would like to buy a single independent house.

Dealer : That'll be difficult because mostly all around here, there are only builder's flats; they build four storeys on an area of 50 or 60 sq. yards.

Customer : No, that is ruled out. The minimum is 100 sq. yards, even if its two storey, I'll buy it. I don't want shared accommodation.

Dealer : What about 150 sq. yards. There is a single storey house for sale in New Lahore Nagar.

Customer : Give me an idea of the rate.

Dealer : Builder's flat of 50 sq. yards will cost you say, 20 Lakhs. But since you're not interested in the, the house what I'll show you will cost you about 70 lakhs. Does that fall into your budget?

Customer : It may, let's see the place first can we go right now?

Dealer : Why not? Let's go what is your good name.

Customer : D.K. Chawla.

Customer : (to the owner) This is Mr. D.K. Chawla, he wants to see your house, Mr. Chawla this is Mr. Mehta.

Mr. Chawla : (Shakes hands and the dealer shows them the house). The house suits me. Shall we talk about the price, I'm ready to pay Rs 65 Lakh, see if you can make the deal.

Dealer : I'll talk to Mr. Mehta, I think he will agree.

Mr. Chawla : Before the deal in finalized. I would like to make few thing's clear first, the house should be free hold and registered in the name of Mr. Mehta. Second, tell me about the stamp duty and other expenses at the time of registry.

Dealer : The circle rates have recently been doubled here, you'll have to pay to the municipal corporation about thirty thousand rupees. Then there is court fee, stamp duty, expenses of deed writers, lawyers etc. the total will come to about more than 1 lakh, pay 1 lakh 20 or 25 thousand.

Mr. Chawla : What about the papers of the house?

Dealer : Oh! They're alright. I have seen them; the house is free hold and registered in the name of Mr. Mehta.

Mr. Chawla : OK then, talks to Mr. Mehta about the price and let me know.

Dealer : Sure, you'll hear from me shortly.

BANK SCENARIO FOR OPENING AN ACCOUNT

A *conversation* demands great *generosity*. On the one hand, it demands the generosity of listening. And perhaps not just of listening but of assuming that the other person is saying something of value, something worth listening to.

Customer : (to a bank employee) Sir, I would like to open a bank account, what is the procedure?

Employee : (gives him an application form) where do you live?

Customer: in Laxmi Nagar.

Employee : Ok, please read this form very carefully. Do you want to open savings or current account?

Customer: Savings.

Employee: Joint or single?

Customer : Single

Employee : Ok, here I'll work the relevant papers. You see two columns here, you'll have to bring a document for each column for address proof, and for example, from this column you can bring an electricity bill or MTNL phone bill. For the other column you can bring your election ID card or driving license or passport.

Customer : How much I'll have to deposit for opening the account?

Employee : Do you want a check book?

Customer : Yes,

Employee : You have to open the account with one thousand rupees. You'll get the check book by post after 10 or 15 days from the date you open the account.

Customer : can I have an ATM card also?

Employee : Why not? Just tick at the relevant column. Like check book, you'll get it after some time.

Customer : (reads the form) It say two witnesses are needed and a person whose account is in this bank.

Employee : Yes, that is very important, a person who has his account here must be known to you. This signature and account number will be needed, witness you can arrange from your neighborhood, after your form is accepted and you have deposited Rs. 1000, and you'll be issued the passbook.

Customer : Thanks, Sir.

Employee : That's alright, fill the form carefully and two photos will be needed, one you have to affix on the form, one will be pasted on your passbook.

Customer : Again thanks, sir.

CHECK DEPOSIT IN BANK

Small talk is used at parties, when meeting people, etc. to be kind and get along with others at the events. Hopefully, small talk leads to more interesting conversations. However, the ability to small talk and use appropriate phrases can help get the conversation flowing.

Customer :	(to clerk) I have just opened an account here and I am new to bank procedures. Could you please tell me how to deposit this check?
Clerk :	It is simple, please take a seat and show me your check. (Seen the check) It's ok, kindly take out a blue colored check deposit slip from that shelf and fill it. There are different slips for demand draft and cash deposit. Have you brought your passbook?
Clerk :	Fill the form, it is easy. Show it to me after filling.
Customer :	(shows him the filled form) right, put your signature over here. You have written the check number. In this number series on the check, the first one is the check number. I have corrected it, now you go to that machine and put your check and this form in that slot. You'll get a photocopy of both from the other right hand slot.
Customer :	Thanks, can you show me the balance in my account.
Clerk :	Yes, give me your passbook well, here it is. For the last fifteen days there has been no transaction in your account.
Customer	shall I have to come here personally to check my account?
Clerk :	For depositing cash or check, you'll have to come but we can send you any transaction in your account by SMS, just give me your cell number.
Customer :	Ok, here it is.
Clerk :	More ever, every month details of your account will be sent to you by SMS.
Customer :	Thanks, if I want to withdraw cash?
Clerk :	You have to fill that white colored withdrawal slip and draw cash from the counter. You must have your passbook with you. It you want to draw more than ten thousand you have to submit a check for that. While writing the check, write 'self' on the line where it is printed 'pay' fill in the amount in words and figure, write your account number and sign it.
Customer :	Thanks again.

CHAPTER 33

A SALESMAN VISITS A HOME

In this type of conversation, a person who is a salesman of a particular company represents his or her company. He/She has to be brief, very clear, confident and fluent in the language he/she speaks so that he/she can convince his/her customers to buy the products of his/her company.

Housewife :	(opening the door after hearing a knock)
Salesman :	Good morning, ma'm, can I have a minute of your time please?
Housewife :	What is it?
Salesman :	Ma'm Phillips is offering 500 Watt mixer and grinder only for Rs. 2,299 there are three jars of best quality stainless steel let me tell you about its functions, this grinding Jar....
Housewife :	It's very costly, we can get such appliances from any other company between Rs. 1500/- and 1900 even for Rs. 1000
Salesman :	Please don't go for local ones or cheap brands, it wouldn't pay in the long run. Philips is a world renowned company; please allow me to come in for a moment.
Housewife :	O.K.
Salesman :	(enters and takes a seat. He unpacks his wares) These are three jars of stainless steel for *chutney*, dry and wet grinding, this mixer can be used for blending, mincing, pureeing and as a juicer. This model offers superior kind of grinding, mixing and whipping protected by drip-safe technology. Also, it has 3 levels of speed.
Housewife :	What about the motor, they usually burn out?
Salesman :	That doesn't happen with Philips. It has a 550W heavy duty motor with and drip-safe technology and detachable blades which can be easily cleaned.
Housewife :	It looks impressive, what discount you're offering.
Salesman :	11% that means you pay Rs. 296 less.
Housewife :	That's not much, still, what about the warranty?
Salesman :	24 months besides you'll be given Rs. 500 worth gift vouchers don't worry ma'm, it is an excellent offer if you can buy right now. Shall I book it for you?
Housewife :	O.k. actually I was in need of a good mixer my old one is worn out can I pay you cash?
Salesman :	Of course ma'm, and thank you.

AT AN NGO [OFFICE OF 'LITTLE ANGELS']

Small talk is used at parties, when meeting people, etc. to be kind and get along with others at the events. Hopefully, small talk leads to more interesting conversations. However, the ability to small talk and use appropriate phrases can help get the conversation flowing.

A young man : (enters) Good morning Alka Didi.

Alka : Good morning Vicky, how are you!

Vicky : Fine, thank you, I would like to meet somebody who can give me more information about this NGO.

Alka : I could gladly help you, still you can meet the founder of this organisation. Enter that room and talk to Mr. Verma.

Vicky : Thanks didi, (enter the room of Mr. Verma) Sir, I joined your esteemed organization a few days ago. I would like to know more about it.

Mr. Verma : I'll be glad to do so. We need young men like you, our Institute gives shelter to abandoned babies and children. There are about 200 of them here. We have a staff of 20 people who look after them.

Vicky : Are the workers paid.

Mr. Verma : Almost no. They can eat and sleep here. But those who come from for away and are very needy, they're paid a little what do you do?

Vicky : I'm doing my graduation, sir.

Mr. Verma : How much time you can put in here?

Vicky : Say, 4 hours, from 4 to 8 p.m. I can manage my studies at night.

Mr. Verma : how did you know about us?

Vicky : From internet, besides, I always had a soft corner for destitute children. I'm fond of teaching also.

Mr. Verma : That is excellent, Vicky. You can invaluably help us. I suppose you can take 50-60 children, make classes, prepare a time table and teach elementary Hindi, English and Maths.

Vicky : I'll do that sir.

Mr. Verma : We lack funds, kindly prepare some matter which can be floated through the internet and in newspapers and magazines. We want to launch this scheme on a war-footing.

Vicky : I'll see to it, can I ask a friend of mine to join?

Mr. Verma : Sure, but he must have a passion for such work as you have. People who simply join to pass time are of little use. We want these children to be nicely brought up and educated. Sometimes I wish that they grow up, graduate, and nicely settle in life. For this we need young and dedicated men like you.

Vicky :	But there are a lot of abandoned and orphaned children. Don't we need more NGO'S.?
Mr.	Verma : Certainly but then there is always paucity of funds. At least we have saved 200 children. They won't become beggars or criminals. There are thousands of such children. I wonder how to save them from that kind of fate. The government and other very rich and powerful individual must come forward. Anyway we should do our best to make our children good and responsible citizens. For this we need a lot of young men and women like you. Talk to all of your friends and other people known to you. We are also in need of clothes.
Vicky :	I'll do my best. I have some rich friends, I'll talk to their family for funds a clothes. In my neighborhood there are some boys who are very good by nature. I'll talk to them about joining our organisation.
Mr. Verma :	That'll be very nice thanks Vicky.
Vicky :	Thank you Mr. Verma for the talk.

A TELEPHONIC CONVERSATION BETWEEN TWO FRIENDS

In a telephonic conversation between two friends, offer a genuine compliment. Try to make it a compliment that involves something they did rather than something they are. This will allow you to carry the conversation forward by asking them about that skill. If you tell someone they have beautiful eyes, they will thank you and the conversation will likely end there, unless you're clever enough to ask them what they do to enhance them.

Neeraj :	Hello Dev, how are you?
Dev :	Oh! Hello Neeraj, how are you my friend?
Neeraj :	Fine
Dev :	So, what gives?
Neeraj :	Nothing new *yaar*. What's happening at your end?
Dev :	I'm with my dad into estate business
Neeraj :	Do you like it?
Dev :	Yes, I like it, I'm learning a lot from dad, and you know he has the Midas touch.
Neeraj :	Yeah, I know thats lucky for you.
Dev :	What're you doing these days?
Neeraj :	Still am hunting for job.
Dev :	Yaar, you have done 2 year diploma course in computer accountancy, any MNC will take you in seconds.
Neeraj :	Yeah, but I'm the ambitions type, you know that. Think high and live high don't you worry; I'll land with a high class job soon.
Dev :	Sure, what about, Samar?
Neeraj :	It is kind of you to remind me of him. If I'm not mistaken, it must be his birthday today.
Dev :	Yes, you seen to be right. Why not go and surprise him?
Neeraj :	Yes, but then he should have invited us.
Dev :	Oh! Come on, it's long since we met him; he might not have even our phone numbers. Let's be generous He's such a nice fellow, mere talking to him is a pleasure.
Neeraj :	That's there, but what present to buy?
Dev :	Oh! We'll buy a bouquet, that's no problem.
Neeraj :	O.k. I think we'll enjoy a lot there, you know he is so fond of Sufi gazal. He used to have a good collection of the CD's.
Dev :	Yes, yes, so far as music is concerned we all three have the same taste.
Neeraj :	Besides we may meet some old friends there. How nice that will be!
Dev :	Really nice, I can't wait any longer, the sun is already setting down. Come straightaway home. We'll both leave together.
Neeraj :	O.k., I'm coming.

BOOKING TICKETS ON PHONE

In this type of telephonic conversation, react to what a person says in the spirit in which that comment was offered.

Customer :	Hello, is it the Delite Cinema?
Employee :	Yes Sir,
Customer :	I'd like to book tickets for the movie 'Singhum.'
Employee :	Which show?
Customer :	7:15 p.m.
Employee :	How many tickets?
Customer :	Four, what is the rate of tickets?
Employee :	Rs. 110 for balcony.
Customer :	What is to be done for booking? Do you need my credit card number?
Employee :	No sir, just tell me your name.
Customer :	S.K. Verma.
Employee :	That's enough, your tickets are booked.
Customer :	From where do I collect my tickets?
Employee :	You can collect them from the ticket counter marked 'Balcony'
Customer :	Thanks
Employee :	It's alright sir.

SALES EXECUTIVE REPORTING TO HIS BOSS

This kind of Conversation is different than a discussion. *A discussion is everyone talking about something.*

Boss :	How did the last week go?
Executive :	Pretty well sir, we had targeted to sell 20 'Pure Water' systems. We sold 14.
Boss :	We fell six short, I can't call it pretty well!
Executive :	My area is Geeta Colony, sir, where about 30 insured people are living. I have a team of four persons; they're working from ten to four. Seeing the locality, I think they have worked well.
Boss :	What about the locality?
Executive :	It's not a posh colony sir, secondly the Jal Board water supply is good and must people have taps. So it becomes rather hard to convince them to spend Rs. 1000 more for better water.
Boss :	The four people working under you, are they sincere?
Executive :	They are, except one, I'll soon replace him.
Boss :	Sales reports from other areas are better than yours. Intensify your efforts.
Executive :	I'll have to increase my staff sir. I have in my mind four busy shopping centre where we can display our 'Pure water' system with catchy slogans like 'Pure water is sure water' with surely of being germ free.
Boss :	I don't think it is a very catchy slogan. I'll provide you with one or two ones, which others are using. Displaying the system in busy areas is a good step, but be sure that smart girls and boys sit there who can offer a convincing talk. You can also arrange make-shift stalls on road side.
Executive :	I'll do that, sir.
Boss :	You may go now, report to me next week with better sale figures.

Chapter 38

TELEPHONIC CONVERSATION AND LEAVING A MESSAGE

In this kind of telephonic talk, you do ask a question that can be answered in a single word, instead of just supplying your own information in response, ask a follow-up question.

Mr. B.K. Gupta :   (on phone) Hello! Can I speak to Mr. Khana?

Receptionist :   May I know who is speaking?

Mr. B.K. Gupta :   I am B.K. Gupta, a friend of Mr. Khana.

Receptionist :   Sir, at the moment Mr. Khana is not in the office.

Mr. B.K. Gupta :   I had to speak to him urgently.

Receptionist :   You can try his mobile, do you have his number, sir?

Mr. B.K. Gupta :   I have tried his mobile, it is coming switched off.

Receptionist :   Quite possible, sir. Actually he has gone to attend an important meeting.

Mr. B.K. Gupta :   I see, I'm going to leave a message with you, please convey it to him as soon as he comes.

Receptionist :   Sure sir, what's the message?

Mr. B.K. Gupta :   Actually we had to meet a friend of ours who is in the hospital. Mr. Khana has to pick me up from my home at 10 a.m. tomorrow. This program stands cancelled as I am leaving for Bombay today. I'll be back within a few days. As soon as I come back, I'll contact him.

Receptionist :   I'll convey the message to Mr. Khana.

Mr. B.K. Gupta :   It's very urgent, please don't forget.

Receptionist :   Rest assured sir, I'll convey the message, and I have already noted it down.

Mr. B.K. Gupta :   Thanks.

COMPLAINT ABOUT MOBILE PHONE BILL

This type of conversation *should be to the point and concise, as well as very official*. One must be firm while complaining, but not rude.

Customer :	(on phone) is it global phone office?
Answer :	Yes, please.
Customer :	I have to make a complaint about an inflated cell phone bill
Answer :	Please locate the customer care number on your phone bill and ring that number.
Customer :	Thanks, (rings customer care number) Hello, I'm Diwakar Rohatgi speaking; it is about my phone bill. The amount is beyond my imagination. Please tell me your phone number and the amount of bill that you have received.
Mr. Diwakar :	My Cell phone number is 9771056756 and the bill amount is Rs. 20,000.
Employee :	Please hold on for a moment. (After a pause) Sir, the bill is alright.
Diwakar :	It's impossible; please connect me to your manager. (Manager on line) Sir, I have received a bill of Rs. 20,000. There is something wrong somewhere. You see I'm an office goer and no businessman. I don't make many calls. My bills are never over Rs. 2000/-. Please get my bill thoroughly checked. Shall I come to you in person?
Manager :	No, It's alright, you'll shortly hear from me.
NEXT DAY	
Manager :	(on phone) Hello! Mr. Diwakar speaking?
Diwakar :	Yes.
Manager :	Sir, your bill has been corrected, It was a computer mistake.
Diwakar :	What's the bill amount now?
Manager :	Rs. 2000/-
Diwakar :	Thanks, please take care that such mistake don't happen is future.

CALLING TO ENTER KBC

This kind of conversation should be brief and one must be very careful and attentive while answering the questions asked by the KBC because the caller may lose a lifetime opportunity!

Mr. B.K. Saxena :	(on an enquiry phone service) I want to take part in KBC could you give me any lead number?
Answer :	We don't have any direct number of KBC, sir. But you can contact Sony Entertainment channel.
Mr. B.K. Saxena :	Please give me their number.
Answer :	Please write down, it is 22430678.
Mr. B.K. Saxena :	Thank you, (rings up Sony) please sir, I want to take part in KBC. Could you tell me the procedure of entering and taking part in the show?
Answer :	Please ring at the number I'm giving and you'll be told the full procedure, or you keep on watching Sony Entertainment Channel we keep giving useful information from time to time.
Mr. B.K. Saxena :	Thanks, first I'll try the phone (ring) will you please tell me the procedure of entering KBC 'Program.
Answer :	Of course, first keep looking filler ads where Mr. Amitabh Bachchan will be asking you the questions, answer the question correctly, the second, you send your answer by SMS or IVR number.
Mr. B.K. Saxena :	Please tell me the numbers.
Answer :	Idea SMS number is 554567 and MTNL landline number is 5052525.
Mr. B.K. Saxena :	When will these questions be asked?
Answer :	Please be on the look out from 27th May onwards. This is the date KBC's 5th audition starts.
Mr. B.K. Saxena :	What happens if I give right answer to Mr. Amitabh's Question?
Answer :	In that case computer will choose candidates. In the first round there'll be 14 thousand people.
Mr. B.K. Saxena :	After that?
Answer :	Computer will again shortlist candidates and if you are lucky you'll be called for audition which has two rounds.
Mr. B.K. Saxena :	It sounds tough.
Answer :	Of course, you'll need lot of luck and talent to succeed.
Mr. B.K. Saxena :	Is that all?

Answer :	No, after clearing the rounds, you'll be tested for the fastest finger round. If you clear it, you'll sit on Hot Seat with Mr. Amitabh Bachchan and play kaun Banega Crorepati Season 5.
Mr. B.K. Saxena :	How much can I win?
Answer :	You can win Rs. One Crore if you rightly answer the first 11 questions and if you give right answer to the 12th question, you will win five crores.
Mr. B.K. Saxena :	Thanks for telling me all this.
Answer :	It's alright. Best of luck.

PLACING ORDERS ON PHONE

In this kind of telephonic talk, react to what a person says in the spirit in which that comment was offered.

Voice :	(in answer to a phone call) McDonalds, sir, what can we do for you?
Answer :	We're having a party, can you send us some dishes, say, in half an hour.
Voice :	Sure sir, where do you want us to deliver?
Answer :	GK II, House Number E 355.
Voice :	Your good name please?
Answer :	P.K. Ahuja.
Voice :	O.k. Mr. Ahuja, what is the order?
Mr. Ahuja :	We want four chicken hamburgers, four vegetable hamburgers, and eight Pizzas.
Voice :	We'll be sending them right away.
Mr. Ahuja :	Thanks; may I know your name?
Voice :	Sunil Mittal at your service, sir.

TELLING THE MANAGER THAT YOU ARE UNABLE TO COME TO OFFICE

This kind of conversation is different than a discussion. A discussion is everyone talking about something.

Dev :   (on phone) Hello, sir! I'm sorry to say, I'll not be able to come to the office today.

Manager :   Why? What has happened, you know we're doing an importance project.

Dev :   Right sir, but my mother has taken ill. I'm with her in the hospital.

Manager :   I see anything serious.

Dev :   It might be. Doctors say an artery carrying blood from heart has hardened. She had complained of severe chest pain we brought her here.

Manager :   It's ok dev. First you look after your mother and if need be, take a few day off. We'll manage here.

Dev :   Thank you, Sir

Manager :   It's alright, God be with you.

CHAPTER 43

CONVERSATION BETWEEN
A COUPLE DURING COURTSHIP

This type of conversation demands the generosity of your own lively intellect, your willingness not just to listen to this other person, but to take what they give, you and move it into a new territory. It's not just a matter of listening, but of giving — and giving wholly of yourself.

Rahul :   (who is waiting in the park, stands up to greet his girl friend Alka) Hello! How are you, please be seated.

Alka :   Late as ever. What is that proverb you quote, 'Better…?

Rahul :   Late than never.

Alka :   (smiles) Tell me, how you are.

Rahul :   Everything fine at this end. My loving, doting parents are worried still about my marriage since the time I told them that I have selected a girl for myself and that they needn't worry.

Alka :   Have you? And who is that lucky girl?

Rahul :   She's sitting right beside me.

Alka :   (blushes) How are you so sure?

Rahul :   Love is the most powerful and most silent of emotions.

Alka :   Please don't grow philosophical.

Rahul :   Shall I grow physical?

Alka :   That kind of talk is downright cheap.

Rahul :   You never let me stay anywhere. Ok, come on, let me take you to a nice place Café Coffee Day, there we can drink, eat and talk a lot. [Inside the cafe]

Rahul :   (to the waiter) Two Cappuccino coffees and noodles. (Looks at Alka, who declines) Ok then a vegetable cutlet a grilled veg-sandwich. Alka, have you seen that film, 'Zindagi Na Milegi Dobara?'

Alka :   Yes, a nice film.

Rahul :   Why don't we see it together and how about seeing it now?

Alka :   Now? Oh! What a nice coffee and what nice cutlets.

Rahul :   My pleasure.

Alka :   I remember that dialogue between Hrithik and Katrina where Hrithik says, "I'm busy today so that I can retire at 40." Katrina says, "How are you sure, you'll live up to 40?" *Today is yours, live it to the full.*

Rahul :	Nice piece of dialogue. Come on Alka; let's see the film together, well, some other time but that dialogue is the crux of the film. Do you follow it?
Rahul :	Do you?
Alka :	Yes.
Rahul :	In what sense?
Alka :	Again you are in a mood to argue. Argument leads nobody anywhere because one is bent upon bringing down one's point whether right or wrong.
Rahul :	Ok, let me ask you one thing.
Alka :	Yes?
Rahul :	I'm in love with you. Is it the same from your side or not?
Alka :	Will you tell me what do you mean by love?
Rahul :	Now, who is arguing?
Alka :	(laughs) No, it isn't that I mean when you love somebody, *it is an unconditional surrender*. You're *caring, respectful* and *full of love*. That's what I think. Your version may be different?
Rahul :	No, it isn't. May I propose to you, on my knees and with a flower in my hand?
Alka :	It isn't necessary. You're such a sweet darling. I'm already in love with you. What about your parents.
Rahul :	They'll be only too happy to accept you once they see you. What's it like at your end?
Alka :	Papa will be in a state of indecision, but should mom put her foot down, he'll have to give in.
Rahul :	Do you think she'll do it?
Alka :	Knowing her, I must say she will. After all, you're to be pronounced as heir to a business, good looking…..(Pronounced 'air').
Rahul :	Please, please enough. I'm not used to hearing my own praise. But things are going to change after marriage.
Alka :	I have inkling.
Rahul :	Well, tell me then.
Alka :	*Heavy words like duty and responsibility creep in*. One's freedom is curbed and often a sense of ownership settles on both the party. Love is almost killed, and quarrels start.
Rahul :	What's to be done then?
Alka :	Don't you worry, as we're aware beforehand, we'll make the most of it.
Rahul :	I'm glad to hear it. Let's leave now.
Alka :	See you tomorrow, Bye!

COLLEGE ADMISSION

Be very attentive, concise and to the point in this type of conversation.

Student :	(enters after being called) Good morning, sir!
Dean :	Good morning. Please be seated. Your name is V.K. Sarswat.
Student :	Yes, sir. Ved Kumar Sarswat.
Dean :	You have applied for B.Com (Hons.)
V.K. :	Yes, sir.
Dean :	Which school did you pass from?
V.K. :	Modern Public School.
Dean :	(reads from transcripts) 90% in aggregate and 94% in commerce, 'impressive'!
V.K. :	Thank you, sir.
Dean :	Why did you choose this college?
V.K. :	Well sir, yours is one of the most reputed Delhi University colleges in North Campus, besides Commerce and Economics Sections are especially good here.
Dean :	How do you know that?
V.K. :	Sir, I have heard from some of my friends who have studied here.
Dean :	Then you must also know that there are a lot of extra-curricular activities.
V.K. :	I know that sir and I'll not disappoint you, I can't say much about sports or athletics but I'm fond of stage, dramatics, debates, etc. I was also the editor of my school magazine.
Dean :	In English, you have good marks. Why didn't you go for that?
V.K. :	Commerce and Economics fascinate me. They're my favourites.
Dean :	You can go now Mr. Sarswat and thanks for coming here. The admission results will be displayed tomorrow.
V.K. :	Thank you, sir.

PRINCIPAL INTERVIEWING CHILD'S PARENTS

This type of conversation demands great generosity. On the one hand, it demands the generosity of listening, and perhaps not just of listening but of assuming that the other person is saying something of value, something worth listening to.

Principal : (to parents) So this is your child. What is your name, son?

Child : My name is Amandeep.

Principal : (smiles) Good. (to parents) You are seeking admission in the Ist grade?

Father : Yes, sir.

Principal : Let me see how he has done in his nursery and K.G. (sees the reports) well! Not bad, there must be other schools in your vicinity. Did you try there?

Mother : There are, sir but please, we would like our child to be admitted here.

Principal : What is your qualifications madam, and are you doing any job?

Mother : I'm an M.A. in English and no, I don't do any job, for me, house job and care of my children comes first.

Principal : I'm glad to hear that, and you sir, what profession you're in?

Father : I work as a Computer Accountant in an MNC.

Principal : I see your salary, please?

Father : Right now, it is Rs. 40,000/- p.m. and increments and other perks are also there.

Principal : That is good. Any other children, you have?

Mother : Her younger sister, Deepa.

Principal : Where is she studying?

Mother : We're still waiting.

Father : Sir, if our son is selected for admission, will she get admission as well.

Principal : (smiles) Will you people have time enough to devote to your child's completion of homework, and regular pursuing of studies which are a must for our school?

Mother : I have all the time apart from my housework. My husband also likes teaching kids.

Principal : Thank you for the interview. You'll hear from us.

INTERVIEW OF A CELEBRITY

A good conversation demands a certain strength — the strength to feel comfortable with someone else; the strength to remain in and of oneself even while being so intent on another; the strength to enter strange, new realms without getting lost. It demands that peculiar posture of poise, leaning neither too far in nor too far back but standing strong while always ready for what may come next.

[Personal Secretary of the film star gestures the waiting reporter to go in.]

Reporter : Good morning, Mr. Ajay Kumar.

Ajay Kumar : Good morning, please have a seat.

Reporter : Thanks.

Ajay kumar : Shall I order something, say coffee.

Reporter : Oh! It isn't necessary.

[Nevertheless he orders two coffees and snacks on phone]

Reporter : Shall we proceed?

Ajay : By all means, shoot.

Reporter : I have heard that you had a humble beginning in a small town. How come you had this tremendously successful journey?

Ajay : Yes, I had a humble beginning I belong to a town in Chhattisgarh. My primary and senior secondary education were completed in the two govt. schools and let me tell you I wasn't good at my studies either (laughs).

Reporting : When did the acting bug bite you?

Ajay : There never was a bug, but a super teacher.

Reporter : Who? Some big film star?

Ajay : No, no, far from it, it was my school teacher who was in charge of my cultural activities. (Pause) You see my only asset was a good appealing face and clear ringing voice, not the baritone of Mr. Amitabh. Out of curiosity, my teacher introduced me to the theatre world and I carried on with it that even surprised me.

Reporter : How did you come to act in films?

Ajay : After school, there were inter-school, and inter-state competitions. At such an event, a film director noticed me. He invited me to Bombay (Mumbai) and well here I'm.

Reporter : Your first film was a hit but then…..

Ajay : (laughs) It was hit by fluke, Later films flopped because I tried to copy Dilip saab and Amitji.

Reporter : How was the situation saved?

Ajay :	I met my old guru who was very happy to see me. He advised me to be my original self without bothering about the outcome. He said, "either be original, your natural self or quit." I never forgot that. He told me some truth which I didn't forget either and that is what made me what I am today.
Reporter :	What truth?
Ajay :	Well what he said was that films are make believe worlds of fantasy and dreams, they are virtual not real, but the more real you are in a film, the better it is. In other words, you must lie very truly, copying, or overacting is of no use.
Reporter :	What are your hobbies?
Ajay :	Reading, sitting on internet and of course, watching T.V.
Reporter :	Your favourite dish?
Ajay :	Home *made daal roti, rajma* and *paneer* dishes.
Reporter :	Very simple, I must say which is your favorite film?
Ajay :	'Gladiator' among many others, '*Bhool Bhuliya*', 'Wanted' and all films of Abbas Mastan.
Reporter :	Your favourite hero?
Ajay :	Besides living legends like Dilip Saab, Amitji, Amir and Salman.
Reporter :	Your favourite heroine?
Ajay :	All are good.
Reporter :	Thad's a diplomatic answer.
Ajay :	(smiles) You better be, where women are concerned.
Reporter :	Your very bad moment?
Ajay :	Yes, I don't know what happened, but once there were *dozens of retakes, when my dialogue carried no punch* and *the face was a dead pan*.
Reporter :	Your best?
Ajay :	When my first film was hit, Me, Mom and Papa, all three of us hugged and wept with joy. I want to seek the blessings of my school *guruji* also.
Reporter :	When do you intend to marry?
Ajay :	Sorry, it is a private matter and not a public one. So no comments. (smiles)
Reporter :	Well thanks a lot, Mr. Ajay, bye!

AN INTERROGATION IN A POLICE STATION

This is a very sensitive conversation. So, react to what a person says in the spirit in which that comment was offered.

[Police inspector and the arrested man V.K. Arora sitting across the table in a police enquiry room.]

Inspector :	What were you doing near Paradise Apartments yesterday night?
V.K. :	Sir, as I have explained to various policemen, I was trying to find a place for peeing.
Inspector :	(angrily hits the table with his palm) Again a lie. Come out with the truth. A constable caught you moving around suspiciously at about 10:30 p.m. there was a murder at that time in paradise apartments.
V.K.'s :	Mouth hangs open in fright. No, sir, I'm innocent I didn't commit any murder.
Inspector :	Every criminal says that now come out with the truth.
V.K. :	Again sir, I haven't done anything. Look, I'm a respectable man. I have never broken law here is my office ID.
Inspector :	So you work in the ministry of agriculture. Anyway, where were you yesterday night between 10 an 10:30 p.m.?
V.K. :	I had a tiff with my wife and in a huff I left the house. I wandered in anger and don't know when and how I came near Paradise Apartments. I had a sudden urge to pee, so as I was looking for a safe place, a policeman caught me.
Inspector :	So you have no alibi to support your statement.
V.K.	Sir, I'm telling you the truth. You can ask my wife about our quarrel. You can ask my neighbours as to what kind of man I am.
Inspector :	We'll do that right now, I am letting you go. A constable will accompany you to verify the truth of your statements. You're not to leave Delhi without the permission of the police.
V.K. :	Thank you, sir.

FATHER SEARCHING FOR A BRIDE
AND TALKING TO A RELATIVE ABOUT IT

This kind of conversation demands the generosity of your own lively intellect, your willingness not just to listen to this other person, but to take what they give you and move it into a new territory. It's not just a matter of listening, but of giving — and giving wholly of yourself.

Shyam Lal :	How are you Hari Kishen!
H.K. :	I'm well but a bit worried.
Shyam Lal :	Why, dear friend?
H.K. :	I have a son aged 30 so far I have been unable to find a suitable match for him.
Shyam Lal :	Why, and what does he do? Isn't his name Rohan?
H.K. :	Yes, he is at a call centre with good salary. I have talked to so many relatives; I have applied through matrimonial ads also but to no avail.
Shyam Lal :	How come?
H.K. :	Sometimes horoscopes don't match, sometimes it is nadi problem. One or two girls we saw but Rohan didn't approve of them nor did we.
Shyam Lal :	I have girl is distant relation will the age of 27 suit you. She lives in Faridabad.
H.K. :	Age is alright.
Shyam Lal :	In that case, I'll let you know further ofter a week.
	[After a week]
Shyam Lal :	I have found out. She has done a computer course after her 12th grade. Her father runs an electric goods shop. She has a younger sister and brother, both are studying.
H.K. :	Does she do a job?
Shyam Lal :	No, her father is of the opinion that her would be in-laws will decide whether she stays at home or does a job.
H.K. :	That's a reasonable outlook. How does she look and whether you know something about her nature.
Shyam Lal :	After my talk with you, I went to Faridabad and observed her. I must say she is good looking and well behaved. She cooks well and is good with children. Almost all children of the neighbourhood gather near her in the evenings she plays with them, tells them stories teaching them, that too free. She is also well read. Prime facie it looks good. What about the horoscope?
Shyam Lal :	There are good hours. I gave them Rohan's bio-data which you had given me. They like the boy and horoscope also matches.

H.K. :	(hugs him out of happiness) You have done a wonderful job, dear friend. You have erased my years of worry, now make a program that we all go and see the girl.
Shyam Lal :	I'll do it shortly, bye now. You'll soon hear from me.
H.K. :	Bye, dear friend and thank you.

CONVERSATION BETWEEN TWO FAMILIES REGARDING MARRIAGE

A good conversation demands a certain strength — the strength to feel comfortable with someone else; the strength to remain in and of oneself, even while being so intent on another; the strength to enter strange, new realms without getting lost. It demands that peculiar posture of poise, leaning neither too far in, nor too far 'back but standing strong' while always ready for what may come next.

Ishwar Prasad : (to his wife) Yesterday Mr. Bhajan Lal's ring came. He said that his family wanted to meet us at least a fortnight before marriage.

Wife : Let's invite them. It's important to discuss certain details before marriage.

I P : Ok, I'll invite them this Friday.

[Both families sitting together over tea, snacks and sweets]

I P : Yes, Mr. Bhajan Lal. Let's talk about marriage arrangements.

B L : Sir, we're parents of the girl, arrangements shall be as you wish.

I P : That is old fashioned Mr. Bhajan Lal, we're on equal footing. Girls and boys share the same plat form these days. What we want is that the money you intend to spend on marriage should be spent in the interest of your daughter.

B L : That's very generous of you. My budget for marriage is Rs. 10 Lakh.

I P : Good, my suggestion is that you spend the minimum on decoration, lights etc. for dinner of baratis, have selected items. It's no use having stalls of all kinds. Before reaching the dinner table, their stomach is full. They fill their plate for dinner but put it into the dustbin half eaten.

B L : I agree with that, quite reasonable.

I P : Please hire a simple band baja and no banquet hall, book a corporation guest house. That way we shall save a lot of money.

I P : Ok, what else.

B L : Nothing much, these are my suggestions, you're free to act as you like. We need nothing. God has given us a lot.

I P : You have left me speechless, we had planned so much to give.

B L : Whatever you want to give, give it to your daughter in cash or kind. Shubham doesn't believe in dowry either.

B L : That's so kind of you, shall we discuss other aspects in details for example, dates of various function, menu for food etc.?

I P : Let's include ladies also in our talk. So where do we start?

Mrs. Prasad : What about the *sagai* date and…..

CHAPTER 50

CONVERSATION AT THE TIME OF ILLNESS

This kind of conversation is different than a discussion. A discussion is everyone talking about something.

Vikram :   (in hospital) How are you feeling Suresh?

Suresh :   I'm afraid it is no good news.

Vikram :   What happened?

Suresh :   The doctor was telling me that there is severe kind of infection in intestines and they may have to operate. The antibiotics and loneliness are almost killing me.

Vikram :   Please don't worry I'm with you. What about the members of your family?

Suresh :   They do come but not often. Father is busy from morning till night. Mother drops in regularly but she can't stay for long.

Vikram :   Other friends must be visiting you.

Suresh :   Yes, but the same thing, they can't stay for long. I feel so lonely and at times, so afraid and depressed.

Vikram :   That's but natural. But don't you be afraid. I have three consecutive holidays coming. I'll be coming to you daily with a friend of mine and we all three will spend long hours chatting, playing cards, listening to music. I'll also bring you my pod, so that in moments of intense boredom, you can have diversion. You have an ear for music, don't you? (Suresh words). Let me talk to your then I'll tell you what it is all this about.

Vikram :   (to the doctor outside) Sir, may I know how long Suresh will be here. I hope he'll get well.

Doctor :   It is some problem in intestines, we are doing the tests. He'll get well don't worry.

Vikram :   But how long will he remain here, doctor?

Doctor :   Nothing can be said with certainty till tests are done.

Vikram :   Thanks doctor, please take care of my friend.

Vikram :   (to Suresh) Don't worry, yaar everything is going to be ok. I have talked to the doctor play cards. It is some mild sort of infection. Come let's play cards.

CHAPTER 51

CONVERSATION BETWEEN A BOY AND GIRL BEFORE ARRANGED MARRIAGE

A good conversation demands a certain strength — the strength to feel comfortable with someone else; the strength to remain in and of oneself, even while being so intent on another; the strength to enter strange, new realms without getting lost. It demands that peculiar posture of poise, leaning neither too far in, nor too far back, but standing strong, while always ready for what may come next.

Ashish : Well! We have been sent here on roof to talk. Shall we proceed?
[Neha keeps silent]

Ashish : Ok, I will start. This is a beautiful moonlit night and I find you here more attractive than when I saw you first. (Neha blushes)

Ashish : Say something, dear. For example, I like you, I love you. Do you also like and love me.

Neha : (pose) Yes.

Ashish : Very well, a big hurdle cleared. Let me tell you about myself. I'm a simple man, I live a simple life. I hate complexities. I don't believe in making big plans and create problem and then solve them. Reading, even writing, watching TV, relaxing over a cup a tea are my best pastime. When I feel a bit lost which I seldom do, I play with my cute nephews and nieces.

Neha : I also like children. They're so innocent and full of curiosity and wonder. You write also?

Ashish : Yes, poems sometimes.

Neha : What kind of poems. Can you recite one?

Ashish : I write when mood takes me on, like when it rains with dark clouds hanging over head or when there is a full moon floating in the sky.

Neha : Why not recite a poem?

Ashish : No, the poem is standing right before me. What's the need? (Neha smiles) What about you?

Neha : I like home, keeping it spick and span, everything in its place. I live to cook food, I like to make purchases for home, but strictly according to the budget. I don't like doing a job. It makes you machine like. When you come home, you're tired, bored and irritated.

Ashish : I'm luckier than I ever thought.

Neha : I don't get you.

Ashish :	When I come home, I like it tidy, clean and a beautiful living, caring wife waiting for me with hot tea ready. This is as far as my ambition goes.
Neha :	Well said anyone would wait eagerly for such a husband.
Ashish :	Anyone? What about you?
Neha :	(laughs) Including, me of course.
Ashish :	(looks into her eyes) Made for each other?
Neha :	(smiles) Seems so.
Ashish :	Nothing doing, say 'yes' or 'no.'
Neha :	Yes.
Ashish :	Well then that settles it. Shall we go home now? Our parents must be waiting.
Neha :	Of course.

SYMPATHETIC CONVERSATION AT THE TIME OF DEATH OF SOMEONE

This kind of conversation is entirely different. One has to be very careful with one's words and gestures. React to what a person says in the spirit in which the comments are offered.

Kanti Prasad : So sorry to hear about the demise of your father really, it's a great loss.

Rajesh : Nobody knew he would go like that (weeps)

K P : Please take heart. What happened?

Rajesh : Father had a history of heart problem, he was walking, talking and suddenly he was no more, he fell down and passed away.

K P : If I remember right, he had a successful heart surgery sometime back.

Rajesh : Yes.

K P : What happened then?

Rajesh : Doctor says that a clot blocked the vein carrying blood to the heart and the death was instant.

K P : What a misfortune.

Rajesh : (breaks down)

K P : Please take hold of yourself. In a short while there is going to be pugree rasam, you'll be the head of the family, so Rajesh, you have to control yourself. (Rajesh keeps silent, brooding)

K P : Rajesh, please snap to of this state. Your father was a great name. Whoever knew him, including me, and had great respect and love for him and the void created by his absence will never be fulfilled. Yet, we have to carry on with the life, do our daily chores and duties

Rajesh : (sighs) Yes; we have to get normal, yet how difficult it is to bear such a loss.

K P : You're right, but take heart. I'm here with you as I always have been, today; even tonight I'll remain with you. Don't you worry? (Rajesh is moved and presses his hand) Small odd domestic jobs, pronounced as 'chores'.

Chapter 53

ENCOURAGING A FRIEND WHEN HE HAS SCORED POOR MARKS

This type of conversation is very different in and unique in itself. One must be very careful with the usage of words, i.e., one should always use sympathetic words and the tone should be soft, yet very inspiring.

Deepak :   What's the matter Nitish, you look so downcast.

Nitish :   Nothing yaar, (pause) but the problem is really. I have scored very poor marks in almost every subject, I almost failed. I shiver to think how I'll face the members of my family.

Deepak :   Yeah, the problem is there but not that big. The solution is to appear again, work hard, and get better marks.

Nitish :   That's there but a year will be wasted.

Deepak :   Does it matter? Life is long and one year doesn't matter much. Time passes all the same whether you pass or fail.

Nitish :   You seem to be right.

Deepak :   In the mean time you can take up any computer one year course in a private computer institution. If I remember right, you're in for computer accountancy in your degree course.

Nitish :   Yes, and come to think of it, I can learn preliminary computer accountancy steps which are addition to my academic studies for reappearing.

Deepak :   That'll be the right thing to do. That way your parents will react in a somewhat difficult way, have the courage to talk to them.

Nitish :   Thanks buddy, you're a real friend.

ASKING LEAVE FROM YOUR BOSS

In this kind of conversation, one should be very brief, to the point and polite.

Boss :   (picks up the ringing phone) Yes?

Ritwik :   I'm Ritwik speaking, could you please grant me leave today.

Boss :   Why do you want a leave, you know how much you're lagging behind in your work schedule. Actually it is all because you take so many leaves.

Ritwik :   You're right, sir, but what shall I do. I keep on ailing and doctors daily write new tests to be done.

Boss :   Ok, you can have it today. What about tomorrow?

Ritwik :   I'll attend the office tomorrow. All the tests are done. It's almost over. Only retests and then diagnosis are awaited. I'll be regular now.

Boss :   It's all right.

Chapter 55

SON ASKING PERMISSION TO MEET A FRIEND

A good conversation demands a certain strength — the strength to feel comfortable with someone else; the strength to remain in and of oneself, even while being so intent on another; the strength to enter strange, new realms without getting lost. It demands that peculiar posture of poise, leaning neither too far in nor too far back, but standing strong while always ready for what may come next.

Son :   Dear Mom, how sweet you are!

Mom :   I see, so you want a favour.

Son :   Why so?

Mom :   When you speak in that special tone of yours, you sure ask for something.

Son :   You're quite smart mom I want to go to Lalit's house.

Mom :   You know I don't want that you should keep his company.

Son :   Why so, Mom?

Mom :   I suspect him to be a rumour monger, it won't take him even a fraction of second to create misunderstanding between two friends or between parents and their children.

Son :   How do you know, Mom?

Mom :   Well I have heard about him and I have seen his shifty cunning eyes. One day he was talking ill of you even to me.

Son :   Oh! Come on Mom, he is a sort of fool, he means no harm. Today is his birthday, let me go please.

Mom :   Ok, for this once only. In future, avoid his company. You know, a person is known by the company he keeps. Widen your friend's circle and choose your friends wisely.

Son :   Thanks Mom. I'll do as you say.

HOW TO FILE AN RTI APPLICATION

This requires to be precise, to the point and technical words. One should aviod being verbose.

Dheeraj :	(to his friend Harish) You have some knowledge of filing RTI, don't you? Kindly guide me.
Harish :	Yes, I'll help you, from which agency you're seeking information?
Dheeraj :	HUDA, Faridabad.
Harish :	Ok, then you take a simple piece of paper and address it to public information officer. HUDA, Faridabad.
Dheeraj :	Is there any format for the letter?
Harish :	No, except that the letter subject should start with 'Request for information under right to information's (RTI Act, 2005." Then you should write your queries point wise.
Harish :	How to close the letter.
Dheeraj :	At the end you have to write the following declaration:
	"I do hereby declare that I am a citizen of India. I request you to ensure that the information is provided before the expiry of 30 day period after you have received the application."
Harish :	Any fee to be deposited and how?
Dheeraj :	The fee varies, for example for departments falling under Haryana Govt. like HUDA, DTCP, etc., it is ₹ 50, for NHAI ₹ 10 only. You can pay it by postal order as it is cheaper then Demand Draft.
Harish :	Any other important points.
Dheeraj :	Yes, right the application and write your postal address send it by registered post and not by couriers.
Harish :	How to find the place for filing and submitting RTI at various places, say in Delhi, Geeta Colony?
Dheeraj :	I think the office is located in the building of Sr. Sec. School, Anand Vihar for complaints against the director of Education. For other departments there must be other places. You can ask some knowledgeable person or try internet or Just – Dial phone enquiry service.
Harish :	Thanks Dheeraj. You have made everything clear.
Dheeraj :	It's alright. After all it is between friends.

ARRIVAL OF A CONSIGNMENT IN BAD SHAPE

It this kind of conversations, one should be precise and at the same times go through all the details.

Secretary :	(to Boss) Sir, there is a phone call from Bombay (Mumbai) from a shipping company.
Boss :	Put me online.
Vice :	This is Columbia Shipping Company. I'm the officer-in-charge of the consignment division. Sir, your consignment has arrived, but I'm afraid to say it is in a rather bad shape. Are you interested to take, delivery, Sir?
Boss :	No, these were electrical lamps and glass shades and they may be fully damaged. So I claim for damages. Anyway thanks for calling, you'll soon hear from us.
Officer :	Thank, Sir.
Boss :	(calls the secretary) Bring me the file of Columbia Shipping Company. Find the consignment note and prepare a claim letter. (Secretary brings file) This is the original consignment note; make a copy of it. Our VAT number is to be quoted on our claim letter. Also please notify the KFL Shipping Services Ltd.
Secretary :	It's better sir, if we call our lawyer. A paper in the file mentions that if we don't take action in time, we will have to pay the damarage charges also while claiming. They'll not pay in full. There are lots of details, terms and conditions.
Boss :	Very well, call Mr. Anand and leave these documents here.

APOLOGISING FOR A MISTAKE TO COLLEAGUES

In this type of conversation, one has to be polite and be able to put across one's thoughts and feelings in an appropriate manner.

Sudhir :   (at his arrival in the office) Hello guys, good morning! How're you.

[There is silence, a few nods]

Sudhir :   Why? What's the matter? Is there something wrong?

A Colleague :   Yes, very wrong.

Sudhir :   What is wrong, my dear Hemant?

Hemant :   What bug had bitten you yesterday? And what grudge do you bear against Krishna?

Sudhir :   Oh that? It was nothing yaar, please don't mind. Just bad mood.

A Colleague :   That would not do. You must apologise for your rude behaviour yesterday.

Hemant :   You talked to none of us, at lunch and you picked up a quarrel with Krishna.

Sudhir :   I'm sorry guys, I was in a bad mood. You know at home, my dad….

Hemant :   We're not concerned as to what happened at your home. Whatever happened, why should you carry it here to the office?

Sudhir :   I'm sorry.

Hemant :   Instead of finding the root cause of your problem and find a solution to it. You come snaking here rude and ready to right.

Sudhir :   Ok, ok, guys, I'm really sorry. It will not happen again. Where is Krishna? Here my friend Krishna, please forgive me for my bad behaviour yesterday. I do apologise to you all sincerely. As penance, I am ready to give special treat to you all with the promise of good behaviour.

Hemant :   I think we should forgive him. After all, it is not daily that he indulges is such odd behaviour (all smile). So what is the special treat?

COMPLEMENTING SOMEONE AT A GET TOGETHER

This kind of conversation demands another kind of generosity, too. It demands the generosity of your own lively intellect, your willingness not just to listen to this other person, but to take what they give you and move it into, new territory. It's not just a matter of listening, but of giving — and giving wholly of yourself.

[A get together party at a house]

Ketan :   Vishal, do you see what a lively person Nikhil.

Vishal :   Yes, he's almost a live wire, bubbling with wit and humor come, let's talk to him.

Both :   Hello, Nikhil

Nikhil :   Oh! Hello, how're you guys.

Ketan :   Well, fine yaar Nikhil, I must say that you're the life of every party.

Nikhil :   Oh! Please don't praise me so much otherwise I'll start bloating like the proverbial frog.

Vishal :   Just tell me how do you manage to be so full of humor and wit, always ready with answers, always so happy an always full of lively and intelligent talk on any topic.

Nikhil :   (laughs) You're at it again well, if you want to know, confidence and being relaxed do the trick to start with, later on you get into the habit of that particular behaviour. By nature also, I'm a happy-go-lucky person. I take things as they come. Why interfere with the cosmic scheme of things.

Ketan :   How I wish I were like you, extrovert, carefree. Honestly speaking Nikhil, I'm your fan to me a party seems colorless without you.

Nikhil :   Thanks for the complement. But it is no use trying to be like somebody. If you're shy or introvert kind, you have to break out of it, but no more lectures. Remember the song 'Don't worry, be happy!'

INVITATION FOR WEDDING

One has to be naturally very polite and formal in this type of conversation. However, if inviting a friend, one can be in formal too!

Harsh :	Hello Punet, how're you?
Punet :	Fine, just as ever, how about you?
Harsh :	Everything is fine. I have good news to tell you. My sister's wedding is going to take place on the coming 18th.
Puneet :	Well that's really good news. Her name is Shilpa, isn't it? A bright young lady, I have seen her twice or thrice at your house. Harsh she completed her MBA and what about the boy.
Harsh :	Take it easy, man. I'll tell you. She has done her MBA and is right now serving as a purchase officer in an international company. The boy has returned from states having done his MD, he is a cardiologist.
Puneet :	A fine match, I must say. How did it all happened?
Harsh :	Actually, my uncle who lives in Bangalore found the match. There were some initial hurdlers, like matching of horoscope, whether Shilpa would work after marriage or not etc., etc. but it all ended fine.
Puneet :	How?
Harsh :	We put some clever pandit on trail for matching horoscope and the boy, his name is Karan, found a job right in Delhi and as such he agreed to let Shilpa do her job. Mind you Puneet, you have to come two days in advance for the marriage. After all, you are my best and closest friend.
Puneet :	Done, I'll be too glad to be of any service to you.

Chapter 61

DISCUSSION ABOUT SOME CURRENT AFFAIRS

A conversation is different than a discussion. A discussion is everyone talking about something.

Darshan :   (to his friend) it is Anna Hazare all over the TV these days, what is your opinion about him and his movement. I fully support him.

Harish :   So do I. I have never seen such mass movement and such massive support for a single person.

Darshan :   Yes, it looks like Gandhi ji's satyagrah a Movement or you can say, Jai Prakash's Movement in eighties.

Harish :   Anna hasn't given in to the government at all. On the contrary, the government is finding it tough to deal with him. The government put 21 conditions in case he goes go on a fast. But team Anna won its first round; it is almost unconditional now the one condition he has agreed to is to go on fast for 15 days.

Darshan :   We owe a lot to Anna Hazare so if the fight against corruption has covered many other things. We owe the RTE facility to him. He won in Bombay (Mumbai) and now it is the turn of Delhi.

Harish :   I was amazed to see people pouring in from almost all states, even school and college students. Three-wheelers, taxi unions all are supporting him.

Darshan :   The reason is his impeccable character and the cause he is fighting for since independence – the most horrible thing that has been happening on large scale shameless, open corruption by politicians, ministers, chief ministers almost everyone without exception.

Harish :   That is why the whole of India and prominent personalities like *Kiran Bedi, Baba Ramdev Swami Agnivesh* among others are with him.

Darshan :   I wonder why did they send him to Tihar? He is no criminal. They could have him or kept him in house arrest.

Harish :   You know he refused to come out of the Tihar jail. Now they're preparing the Ram Lila ground for him where he will fast. Bomb squads and sniffer dogs are there. Dr. Trehan is checking Anna Hazare's health. By God's grace, he is doing fine now.

Darshan :   I think his main strength is that he talks simple, direct and straightforward. He is very right when he says that prices are rising because of corruption. People are just sick of corruption.

Harish :   Do you think, Anna will succeed in his mission?

Darshan :   I think so, the Lokpal Bill should be introduced and passed, or Anna will begin his 15-day fast from the Ram Lila Maidan tomorrow.

Harish :   God bless Anna. Let's also go to the Ram Lila Maidan.

CONGRATULATING SOMEONE FOR DOING WELL IN THE EXAMINATION

In this kind of conversation, one should be very spontaneous, encouraging and lively. One must also know to use the right words that fit the occasion.

Latika : Hai Charu! Congrats, you have passed with flying colors.

Charu : (smiles) Thanks.

Latika : Tell me your aggregate and how much you have scored in your favorite subject.

Charu : Aggregate is 96 p.c. and in English it is 98 p.c.

Latika : I have never heard about such high score in a subject like English.

Charu : There have been cent percent results also.

Latika : I knew you were a brilliant student, still such achievement is stupendous, brilliant, great.

Charu : Hold it, Latika, enough of adjectives.

Latika : Tell me the secret of your success.

Charu : Oh nothing yaar. God has been kind to me and given me the power to focus with a sharp memory. I once read and don't forget. I hope I'm not blowing my own trumpet. May be lady luck was smiling on me.

Latika : Anyway, please accept my heartiest congratulation again. What rare your future plans? Why not aim for IAS exams?

Charu : You know my favorite subject. I'll prefer to be a lecturer in English and that too god willing, in Delhi University.

Latika : You know you'll need some connections for that.

Charu : My English lecturer sir Ganpati has been very kind and co-operative with me so far. He has encouraged me to do B.A. English humors. There a, if my result is good, he has promised to help me.

Latika : That is great drop home some time, mom has specially invited you.

Charu : I'll be glad to come.

LANDLORD AND TENANT CONVERSATION

One should be precise, to the point and careful with one's words in this kind of conversation.

Tenant : (opens the door after hearing the knock) Good morning Kashyap Saheb. Please come in.

Mr. Kashyap : How are you Mr. Dev! (Jokingly) Are you taking good care of my house?

Mr. Dev : Of course sir, please look for yourself, and after all we live here.

Mr. Kashyap : Yes, that's there. Let me see it. Why this dampness in kitchen wall? It's quite an old complaint.

Mr. Dev : You see sir, the people living upstairs are rather careless. Some amount of water is always there in their kitchen under the sink area because the slope is not right.

Mr. Kashyap : Have you talked to them?

Mr. Dev : Many times but no use.

Mr. Kashyap : I know a mason, he is a good one and an expert in dealing with such problems. I'll send him here & he'll do the needful of course you have to pay him the house also needs painting.

Mr. Dev : I'll have it painted next month.

Mr. Kashyap : The rest seems ok. Are you paying the maintenance charges of society regularly?

Mr. Dev : Yes, sir, I take care of that won't you sit down and have a cup to tea.

Mr. Kashyap : No, thanks, I'm rather in a hurry. I'm sorry to say, but one of your cheques has bounced.

Mr. Dev : I know and I rather feel ashamed. Some unexpected expenditure came. Would you like to be paid in cash right now?

Mr. Kashyap : That will be good. But be careful in future.

Mr. Dev : Yes, sir. It'll not happen again.

Chapter 64

AN ELDERLY PERSON TEACHING HIS GRANDSON ABOUT LIFE

A good conversation demands a certain strength — the strength to feel comfortable with someone else; the strength to remain in and of oneself, even while being so intent on another; the strength to enter strange, new realms without getting lost. It demands that peculiar posture of poise, leaning neither too far in, nor too far back, but standing strong while always ready for what may come next.

Grandpa : Hello, son how are you!

Grandson : I'm very well grandpa. It has been many days since you told me a story.

Grandpa : An, son! You're grown up now. I'll tell you something different today.

Grandson : What's that grandpa?

Grandpa : That's about life. Life is to be lived and not to be spent.

Grandson : Meaning?

Grandpa : Meaning enjoy life, don't carry it like a burden. For this you must take care of a few things.

Grandson : What are they?

Grandpa : First you should decide what you're going to become in life and then put your whole energy into achieving that goal.

Grandson : I want to become a doctor.

Grandpa : That's good, just stick to it. Next, learn to handle money earn more, save even more and spend less.

Grandson : Why grandpa? I want to buy so many things.

Grandpa : Exactly, things are so many and money is always limited, so you should be discerning, wise and choosy. You aim to become a doctor?

Grandson : Yes

Grandpa : You'll be treating patients but you must first learn to be patient yourself.

Granson : Please explain.

Grandfather : Patience always pays. Nothing happens at once. Hurry and worry are a course of modern life. Avoid them and avoid short cuts.

Grandson : I'm hungry grandpa; I want a cake and burger.

Grandpa : I'll offer you salad and juice instead. Don't go for soda or cola drinks and junk food. They're addictive. Eat nutritious and cooked food and lots of fruits. Eat well and dress well always.

Grandson :	What's that?
Grandpa :	A man is known by the company he keeps. After parents it's the company that counts avoid bad boys who bunk classes, smoke or wander aimlessly. Tell me about your friends.
Grandson :	They're all good grandpa. You have said it to me before also. I'm careful about that and most of my friends are known to you.
Grandpa :	That's good, one more thing before you feel bored. Lead a balanced life.
Grandson :	Explain grandpa
Grandpa :	Lord Buddha laid great emphasis on Samyak marry or middle path which he also called golden path. Excess of everything is bad, even goodness in excess may prove bad.
Grandson :	How so?
Grandfather :	Well if you're too good, people will misuse your gentleness and exploit or cheat you. So avoid extremes in any matter. Have you read about Darwin?
Grandson :	Yes.
Grandfather :	Then you should know about survival of the fittest. Only the strong survive, rest perish. Be strong in mind and body be fully aware of yourself and your surroundings, it is a bad habit to be lost in thoughts. Your mind should be where your body is. Do everything with great awareness and sharp focus. Ok? Digest.
Grandson :	I'll grandpa, you're so good and I love you so much (kisses him). I'll always be aware of what you said today or what you may say in future.

Chapter 65

WAITER TAKING AN ORDER AT A TABLE IN A RESTAURANT

This talk or conversation should be polite, precise and one must be very careful with the words, one uses, ie, a waiter should be very formal and polite to hsi customers. Similarly, the customers should also be well-mannered.

[Mr. Gupta in a restaurant with family]

Mr. Gupta :	(gestures to a waiter) Water for all please.
	[After drinking water, Mr. Gupta and family read the menu cards, handed over to them by waiter]
Mr. Gupta :	Any special dish of your restaurant today?
Waiter :	Yes sir, *Karhai daal* and *Paneer Koftas*.
Mr. Gupta :	Good, one plate of each, we would like to taste it first.
Waiter :	(writing on note pad) what else sir?
Mr. Gupta :	(to children) what will you two girls have?
Khushi :	*Shahi Paneer* for me.
Muskan :	*Dam Aloo* for me.
Mr. Gupta :	(to waiter) half plate of each, you papa and mom?
Papa :	*Palak Paneer* for both of us.
Mr. Gupta :	(to waiter) two plates of palak paneer one plate aloo mutter and one plate curry. To begin with bring tomato soup for each of us.
Mrs. Gupta :	One plate of *Raita* and *Rice* also.
Muskan :	Onions and pickle also.
Mr. Gupta :	Oh *Beta*, they serve it free, you'll get papads also.
Waiter :	What about *Chapattis*, sir?
Mr. Gupta :	Yes, two *Laccha Paranthas*, two *Roomali Rotis* and two *Missi Rotis*. That's all.
	[After dinner]
Waiter :	What would you like for dessert, sir?
Mr. Gupta :	*Gulab Jamuns* for each and thanks for the prompt service. Bring the bill, as well.

A BUSINESS CALL, FIXING A MEETING WITH AN OFFICIAL TO SEAL A DEAL

In this kind of conversation, one should be precise, formal, to the point and careful with the words one uses.

Mr. Arora (Client) : Hello Mr. Sandeep how are you?

Sandeep (Architect) : I am fine Mr. Arora.

Mr. Arora : Can we meet some time tomorrow; I wish to discuss our upcoming project with you.

Sandeep : Tomorrow shall be difficult for me; by the way what project is it?

Mr. Arora : This time it is a big one. It is a group housing project with 500 dwelling units and we are in a hurry. So try to make it tomorrow.

Sandeep : As I told you tomorrow is difficult, one of my dear clients like you is coming to meet me all the way from Dubai.

How about, day after tomorrow?

Mr. Arora : That suits me, what time?

Sandeep : 11 a.m. at my office!

Mr. Arora : Not eleven, I have to attend my kid's school function, I shall be free by 12:30 p.m. we can meet at lunch if it suits you.

Sandeep : By all means, will wait for you at lunch. Do let me know what you would like to eat.

Mr. Arora : South Indian food, from the famous shop across the street.

Sandeep : Great see you day after tomorrow then.

A CLERK IN MEETING WITH A CLIENT

In this type of conversation, the clerk has to be clear, concise and assertive in his talks to convince and influence his/her client or customer. Similarly, the cilent also has to be polite and careful of the words he/she uses.

Ajay (Client)	Good Morning Ankit!
Ankit (Clerk)	Yes sir, how may I help you?
Ajay :	I wish to transfer some money for my brother in UK.
Ankit :	Sure sir, please have a seat.
Ajay :	Thanks.
Ankit :	Do you have an account in our bank?
Ajay :	Yes.
Ankit :	Please tell me your name and account number.
Ajay :	Ajay Verma, Account Number APN0035987651234.
Ankit :	Give me a minute, let me open your account details on computer.
Ajay :	Sure.
Ankit :	What is the purpose of this remittance?
Ajay :	Education.
Ankit :	Sir does your brother have an account in a UK bank?
Ajay :	He reached there just 15 days ago; he does not have any bank account. I plan to transfer money to one of his colleague's account.
Ankit :	Then you will have to show it as gift.
Ajay :	That's fine; I have to send just 500UK Pounds.
Ankit :	Ok but one more problem, your account is just one month old, you need at least one year old account for such remittance or produce a one year statement of some other bank account where you hold an account for more then one year.
Ajay :	Oh man! That is ridiculous, you people promise all possible services when you want us to open an account in your bank and this is what happens when we actually need your service.
Ankit :	Sir try to understand, we have to abide by the rules of the bank.
Ajay :	Thank you so much for your time, I will try my other bank account and make sure that I close my account here.

CHAPTER 68

BOSS GIVING INSTRUCTIONS TO HIS SECRETARY

This conversation should be brief, to the point and commanding as far as the boss is concerned, and the secretary should be attentive and courteous, while listening and answering.

Secretary :	Good Morning Sir, did you call me?
Boss :	Yes Arti, but make a habit to bring pen and writing pad every time, I call you.
Secretary :	Sorry Sir, I will be back in minute.
	(She goes back to bring pen and paper)
Secretary :	Yes Sir!
Boss :	Note down a few tasks you have to do within this week - Take my mobile phone and try to transfer all the contacts on computer. Make an elaborate contact list segregating clients, friends, vendor's consultants, office staff, suppliers etc.
Secretary :	Ok Sir!
Boss :	This list should have a title, contact name, phone number, email id, address, office and land line number etc.
Secretary :	Ok Sir!
Boss :	I need this because when I need to talk to somebody, all I need to give you is some reference and you should be able to give any contact information of that very reference immediately.
Secretary :	Ok Sir!
Boss :	Hope you clearly understood what I mean.
Secretary :	Yes Sir!
Boss :	Arti this document should remain confidential and not to be shared by anyone.
Secretary :	Yes Sir!
Secretary :	May I leave sir?
Boss :	One more thing, we feel office expenditure is going up day by day, I want you to make a list of monthly expenses this time and discuss it with me at the month end so as to where we can cut down the costs, and I want all staff to be part of this discussion.
Secretary :	Ok Sir, I will do that and keep you informed.
Boss :	Thanks, you may carry on with your work now, and connect me to Mr. Rajeev from Western Developers.
Secretary :	Yes Sir.

DEVELOPER, ARCHITECT & CONTRACTOR AT A CONSTRUCTION SITE

This is a business or official talk and one must be careful of the usage of words. Generally, one should be very concise and to the point.

Anil (Developer) : Vijay & Arun, I want both of you to assess the site conditions once again since I doubt that the designs we have made should result in cost effective construction.

Vijay (Architect) : Anilji I disagree with you on this one, I agree that the site has lot of contours, but we have worked on a lot of permutations and combinations before finalizing the present design.

Anil : Vijay, I do not doubt the hard work & capabilities of your team, but instead of making the building blocks on the sloping portions of the site, why not use the flat pieces, so that the construction is fast and economical.

Arun (Contractor) : Anilji and me, as designers we have to strike a balance between aesthetics and cost keeping in mind the existing parameters. In this particular case, placing building blocks on contoured parts of land shall result in a very unique look of building, enhancing the character of the resort.

Anil : What about the increased cost and time factor?

Vijay : Might be a bit expensive and will take couple of months longer but right from the start you told us that this building should become an address, a landmark….! And you approved the three dimensional view also.

Arun : Anilji, I think Vijay has a point too.

Anil : Ok guys, what I request is, do a small working on the cost and give me an analysis of it and the time difference involved if we are to go for the present scheme.

Vijay & Arun : Ok, sounds fine to us.

Anil : Ok, see you next Monday, we shall take the final decision, the same day.

WANTING TO PAY TAXES AT THE GOVERNMENT DEPARTMENT

This talk has to be very polite, official, brief and to the point.

Kunal :   Sir, I wish to pay Income tax, could you help me with certain queries?

Clerk :   Sure go ahead.

Kunal :   Should TDS be applicable on the entire invoice value or is it only on Professional fee excluding Service Tax?

Clerk :   TDS shall be applicable on full bill value.

Kunal :   Sir I want to know about deduction of TDS on professional services taken from foreign consultants and how much rate of TDS is applicable.

Clerk :   Specify the country and the exact nature of services rendered by consultant. But normally TDS is deductible @ 10.5575% if the foreign party as Pan, and 20% if it doesn't have a PAN.

Kunal :   We are a design consultancy company, we do Interior designing with execution (Material and labour) we have just paid service tax, do we have to pay any other tax too?

Clerk :   Execution of contracts could be under works contract wef 1.6.2007. prior to that, no levy. Composition applicable – or period 1.6.2007 to 1.3.2008 + 2.06% ST and thereafter 4.12% on receipt of money basis. Interest on delayed payment is 13%.

Kunal :   Thank you so much for your help.

Clerk :   You are welcome.

TELEPHONIC ENQUIRY

This conversation has to be very subjective and depends upon the type of enquiry you have to make. Nonetheless, one has be very polite, precise and to the point.

Voice :   (on phone) Can I speak to Mr. Nagpal please?

Answer :   He is not here at the moment. May I help you?

Voice :   I gave an interview last week. I'd like to know the result. May I know who is speaking?

Answer :   I'm vineeta, Mr. Nagpal's secretary. May I know your good name, the post which you applied for and the date of interview?

Voice :   My name is Venugopal. I applied for the post of computer operator and I was interviewed on the 7th of this month.

Vineeta :   Please hold on for a moment Mr. Venugopal, let me check. (Pause) you have been shortlisted for the next round which will take place, on the 21st of this month.

Venugopal :   Thanks, Ms. Vineeta.

Chapter 22

GIVING INTERVIEW FOR A PSU

A 'PSU' stands for a Public Sector Unit. This is an interview, so the candidate has to be polite, brief and precise while answering only the questions that has been asked and avoid talking anything extra or frivolous.

[Candidates waiting to be interviewed for Probationary Officer's Post at SBI]

Peon :	Mr. K.C. Chawla
K.C. :	Yes, please
Peon :	Go in please
K.C. :	(knocks and enters three persons are sitting in the interview board) Good morning gentlemen.
1st Member :	Good morning Mr. Chawla, please sit down. Your full name?
K.C.	Keshav Chandra Chawla.
2nd member :	(looks at papers) Mr. Keshav, what made you interested in a bank job? You have done well in your exam.
K.C. :	Thanks Sir. I like responsible and challenging jobs sir.
3rd member :	You mean to say other jobs carry no responsibility.
K.C. :	Of course they do, sir some even more but a bank is a powerful place because it deals with the most powerful commodity money. A bank is where money is.
2nd member :	If you're appointed what kind of post would you like to hold and why?
K.C. :	A post like that of PRO. I like to help people with their difficulties, guide them instruct them in any and every way. You know sir, our paper work is so ardors and so long.
3rd member :	But rulers are to be strictly adhered to.
K.C. :	Yes, sir but seeing the age and circumstances of a person some minor things can be overlooked.
1st member :	How do you think a good bank should operate?
K.C. :	In my humble opinion sir, there should be more transparency. More polite and helpful talk, more staff and subsequently no long queues. A bank should earn good money and give quality service to its clients; we should never less our patience or temper. Smart dressed people and smart counters help a lot.
3rd member :	(smiles) Good, try that when you are in service. Any more suggestions Mr. Chawla?
K.C. :	Please sir, I was only giving my humble views, don't take it otherwise. May be I talked too much.
1st member :	It's alright Mr. Chawla. You'll be informed about the result next week. You can go now.
K.C. :	Thank you, gentlemen.

A COACH TALKING TO HIS PLAYERS BEFORE A CRICKET MATCH

In this kind of conversation, one, i.e., the coach in this case, should be very inspiring and encouraging to his players and should be very precise and to the point. The players, on the other hand must be polite and attentive towards their coach..

Coach : (to team prior to a match) we'll soon be entering the 3rd round for the Ranji Trophy. The opposite team is very strong so I want all of you to be aggressive right from the beginning.

One player : You know my problem sir, the moment I begin to hit, I'm usually caught out.

Coach : Yeah, that's there I'm sorry to say that your lift strokes lack poser, it would be better if you keep a low profile, that way more runs can be scored. You're an expert in hitting the ball in right direction between spaces. So don't lift, keep the ball to ground. (Looks at another player) You avoid your left hand drives. It has not paid so far. I have nothing to say to Vishal, he is a brilliant player. Ketan and Swami you'll be at the tail end. Your specialty is bowling and not batting.

One player : It seems a cloudy today. Sudden darkness and brightness sometimes result in wrong judgement of the direction of the oncoming ball.

Coach : That is right there is only one solution for that. Even otherwise it is a first class strategy. as I have told you many times also, keep your eyes glued to the oncoming ball, if you can do that then if the ball is straight you can drive it in any direction, even for fours & sixes. If it is a dangerous googly, you can be on defense. Any more doubts or questions?

[Silence]

Then play and play, as if your life depends on victory.

A TEACHER TEACHING IN THE CLASS

This type of conversation is very exclusive and different. The teacher has to be very clear, subjective and precise. At the same time, he/she should be able to make the subject simple and interesting to the students. The students also have to be very attentive and polite to their teacher.

Teacher :	Our today's topic is articles which are three in number, namely a, an and the. They are used before nouns. A and an are called indefinite articles while the is known as definite article.
One student :	Sir, why are they called definite and indefinite?
Teacher :	A and an are used for any noun which is one in number. For example, (writes on blackboard) I saw a dog. Now it can be any dog, not a definite one. But if you refer to the same dog again and say (writes on black board) the dog was black in colour, then it becomes a definite dog because it has already been referred to.
Another student :	What is the difference between the use of a and an, sir?
Teacher :	There are 26 alphabets in English language, 21 consonants and five vowels namely a.e,i,o,u. (writes on blackboard) A word that begins with a vowel sound, say, egg, will take an and not a before it, e.g., an egg.
Another student :	But we say an hour, sir. Why? It is a consonant.
Teacher :	Good question, but you didn't listen to me carefully. I said a word that begins with a vowel sound and not vowel. (Writes) That is why we say –an honest man, an inkpot, an heir which is pronounced as air.
Another student :	Where do we use the sir?
Teacher :	It is a long list but I'll mention some important ones. We use the before the names of rivers, sea, oceans mountain ranges, islands, countries with plural names, scriptures etc. we don't use the before proper nouns. That's all for today.

BOY PROPOSING TO A GIRL ON A DATE

This kind of conversation demands a special type of generosity requires the generosity of your own lively intellect, your willingness not just to listen to this other person, but to take what they give you and move it into a new territory. It's not just a matter of listening, but of giving — and giving wholly of yourself.

Devan :	Hello Reema, how are you!
Rima :	Fine, how are you!
Devan :	Fine, happy. Do you know why?
Rima :	Why?
Devan :	Because I'm always relaxed in your company.
Rima :	(feels happy but doesn't show) What is there in my company?
Devan :	Something mystical, beyond explanation.
Rima :	Do you intend to stay here in the park all the time?
Devan :	Oh! No. I'm sorry, it's getting hot; let's go to our favourite joint, Barista.
Devan :	(to waiter) Two espressos, a cheese and a veg hamburger, anything else dear?
Rima :	No, that'll suffice.
Devan :	You know something, Rima?
Rima :	What?
Devan :	I see oceans in your eyes.
Rima :	Come on, you know such talk upsets me.
Devan :	Why?
Rima :	It is romantic and we're just friends.
Devan :	Many times friendship is just a stepping stone to romance.
Rima :	Do you feel that way?
Devan :	Yes, what about you?
	[Keeps silent but amused]
Devan :	(in a far away voice) Rima, can you see the floating moon through this glass wall?
Rima :	Yes.
Devan :	Shall I ask the manager to dim the lights further, I'll be so wonderful. I think many couples sitting here would welcome it.
Rima :	(smiles) Go and try.
	[Lights are dimmed]

Devan :	(sighs) Ah! Its sheer magic, this shaded brilliance of moonlight. I wish to say something to you. The moment is right.
Rima :	You have wished to say something so many times but have never said anything?
Devan :	I thought people were telepathic.
Rima :	What?
Devan :	Oh! Forget it. What I always wanted to say but could not say was and is 'I love you and will you please marry me.' (Laughs)
Rima :	Do you think it is laughing matter?
Devan :	(sorely) No, I'm sorry. I'm very serious, I simply laughed at the absurdity of my proposition. Rima, please, do you accept me and my love?
Rima :	(after a pause) Yes. Truly speaking, I like you Devan and love you as well, but at times your eccentricities upset me.
Devan :	Nobody is perfect. But it is acceptance that solves all matters. We're in love that is the great thing shall we more how and talk to our respective parents.
Rima :	Ok! Let's go.

CONFESSION TO FATHER IN A CHURCH

This kind of conversation takes place only in churches. In this, the ones who confesses has to be clear, concise and polite. The Father (priest), on the other hand, thus to be very attentive, living and caring in his talks.

[A man is kneeling in confession in a church. There is a partition between him and the priest or father, who is listening and talking to him.]

Man :	I have gravely sinned father, please forgive me. My soul is restless, I cannot sleep without tablets and through out the day guilt is eating into me like a worm. I am rich powerful but it is of no consolation.
Father :	What have you done? Speak to me, child without fear for you are in the house of God. Nobody is a sinner here and it is not for me to judge you. Power of judgment rests with God. So, speak.
Man :	I have betrayed my friend in money and in love.
Father :	Go on, talk son.
Man :	We were childhood friends, we established a business together. The business ran well but I developed a weakness for my friend's wife. She knew it. She showed neither favor nor disfavor. When I was deeply involved with her, she asked me for money. I gave her what she asked for but soon I couldn't meet her demands, so I bungled the accounts of my friend.
Father :	Where is she now?
Man :	She has left both of us and my friend is bankrupt. Betrayed by me, he is in a shocked state in a hospital.
Father	Are you married, son.
Man :	Yes and my wife is also grief stricken. I just don't know what to do. It is all confusion, chaos and misery.
Father :	Peace be onto you son. Since you have confessed, I forgive you in the name of God. Don't sin again. Do penance. Ask for forgiveness from your wife and you friend; compensate him for the financial loss you have caused. Take care of him in the hospital till he recovers.
Man :	(sobs) Oh! Father forgive me forgive me please.
Father :	Amin! Go in peace son for God has forgiven you.

CHAPTER 22

GOING TO THE CHEMIST AND ASKING FOR MEDICINES

In this type of Conversation, the customer/buyer has to be polite, clear and to the point as to what he/she requires. The chemist, on the other hand has to very polite, attentive and careful of the words, he/she uses while dealing with the customers.

Customer :	Can you give me these medicines? (Hands him over a paper)
Chemist :	No sir, these are schedule L drops which can't be given without a physician's prescription you can't buy them OTC.
Customer :	What's OTC?
Chemist :	Over the counter. Certain drops like pain killers, some antibiotics, stomach and headache or digestion medicines you can buy right away.
Customer :	What about the medicines I have showed you.
Chemist :	(Reads from the paper) These are zolfresh 10 mg. pehil .5 me serevace.25. These are all medicine concerned with mind for sleep depression and anxiety disorders. No chemist will give these to you without medical prescription.
Customer :	I see. Actually I lost the prescription. Then I phoned the doctor. he named the medicine and I wrote them down.
Chemist :	Please go to the doctor again and have them prescribed.
Customer :	Ok, but you can give me Crocin and Zintec.
Chemist :	Sure, how may?
Customer :	Five each. Also give me some good cough syrup.
Chemist :	Take Benadryl, it is a good one, cures all sorts of throat disorders. You can have pack of Novaclox as well, it is an antibiotic but better consult a doctor for it.
Customer :	Thanks, give me the syrup and tablets, the rest I'll get prescribed.

Section 4
Vocabulary

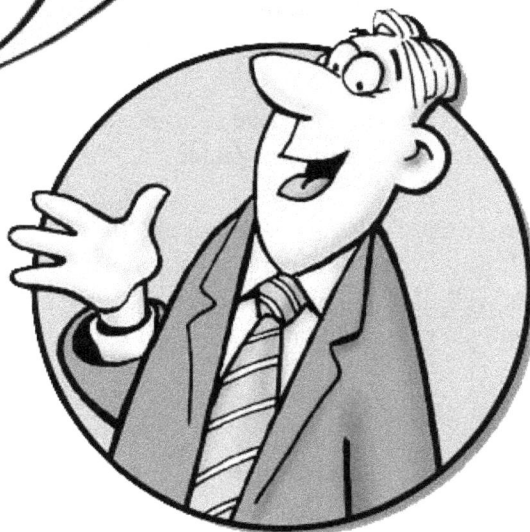

CHAPTER 1

BUILDING A BETTER VOCABULARY

Everyone from the beginning -- learners in English to veterans in journalism know the frustration of not having the right word immediately available in that lexicon one carries between one's ears. Sometimes it's a matter of not being able to recall the right word; sometimes we never knew it. It is also frustrating to read a newspaper or homework assignment and run across words whose meanings elude us.

Language, after all, is power. When your children get in trouble fighting with the neighbours' children, and your neighbours call your children, little twerps and you call their children, nefarious miscreants— well, the battle is over and they didn't stand a chance. Building a vocabulary that is adequate to the needs of one's reading and self-expression has to be a personal goal for every writer and speaker.

Reading Magazines, Journals & Newspapers to Enhance Your Vocabulary

Using some durable piece of paper or the insides of the ripped-off covers of old notebooks—begin to write down words in small but readable script that you discover in your reading newspapers, magazines and journals which you can't define. Read as many journals, magazines and newspapers that challenge you in terms of vocabulary. Pursue words actively and become alert to words that you simply overlooked in the past. Write down the words in one column; then, later, when you have a dictionary at your disposal, write down a common definition of the word; in a third column. Now write a brief sentence using the word, underlined.

Carry this paper or cardboard with you always. In the pauses of your busy day—when you're sitting on the bus, in the dentist's office, during commercials—take out the paper and review your vocabulary words until you feel comfortable that you would recognise (and be able to use) these words the next time you see them.

The amazing thing is that you will see the words again—even "nefarious miscreants," and probably sooner than you thought. In fact, you might well discover that the words you've written down are rather common. What's happening is not that, all of a sudden, people are using words you never saw before, but that you are now reading and using words that you had previously ignored. This is the easiest way to develop and enhance your Vocabulary in English or in any other language.

What are the prime ingredients of English Vocabulary?

Basically the English Vocabulary consists of *Prefixes and Suffixes, Antonyms and Synonyms, Homophones and Homonyms, Idioms, Proverbs and Phrases, One-Word Substitutes, Acronyms and*

Abbreviations, etc. All these topics have been discussed properly and explained thoroughly in the subsequent chapters that follow.

There are multiple exercises based on different topics in order to increase the word knowledge on a wider scale. Each topic has a different exercise with a description given before it as to how to go about it, the relevant words and meanings associated with the exercise and all the necessary details needed. The standard remains generalised for everyone to access the book and make good use of it, and this is in fact, the Basic Aim of the Book.

CHAPTER 2

ANTONYMS

The word, 'antonym' was coined in the 19th century by the philologists. The word, antonym comes from Greek, *anti (opposite)* and *onoma (name)*. This suggests that antonyms are words which have opposite meanings. The term, 'antonym' is synonymous with opposite. Antonyms tend to be *adverbs*, *adjectives* and *verbs* with relatively few nouns. Words opposite to each other may be similar in most other respects. One word may have more than one antonym.

Generally, our day to day English Vocabulary consists of antonyms and in order to improve one's vocabulary one needs to be familiar with them as they play an important role in helping to build a strong base of English.

For example:

An antonym for 'behave' would be 'misbehave'. Similarly, the opposite or antonym for 'agree' would be 'disagree'.

Inside – Outside

Balance – Imbalance

Dependent – Independent, etc.

EXERCISE

The following exercise provides the reader with a list of words given with two options each. The reader needs to select the right antonym out of the two choices to get the correct answer.

1) Overwrought
    a) agitated   b) calm

2) Contemptuous
    a) disdainful   b) respectful

3) Zeal
    a) apathy   b) fervour

4) Jagged
    a) smooth   b) spiky

5) Loyalty
    a) allegiance   b) treachery

6) Just
    a) unfair   b) fair

7) Guilty
    a) culpable   b) innocent

8) Rabble
    a) mob   b) nobility

9) Prone
    a) vulnerable   b) resistant

10) Lack
    a) abundance   b) deficiency

11) Adhere
    a) detach   b) separate

12) Alienate
    a) harmonise   b) patriotism

13) Adversity
    a) prosperity   b) accuracy

14) Acquit
    a) convict   b) innocent

15) Intentional
    a) accidental   b) deliberate

16) Optimist
    a) pessimist   b) opportunistic

17) attractive
    a) repulsive   b) compulsive

18) Abundant
    a) immense   b) scarce

19) Captivity
    a) imprisonment   b) liberty

20) Transparent
    a) translucent   b) opaque

Answers

1) Calm	2) Respectful	3) Apathy	4) Smooth	5) Treachery
6) Unfair	7) Innocent	8) Nobility	9) Resistant	10) Abundance
11) Detach	12) Harmonise	13) Prosperity	14) Convict	15) Accidental
16) Pessimist	17) Repulsive	18) Scarce	19) Liberty	20) Opaque

Choose and tick the correct antonyms of the following words from the options given below the words.

1) Deterioration
   a) improvement   b) depletion

2) Erratic
   a) irregular   b) consistent

3) Factitious
   a) genuine   b) improper

4) Boisterous
   a) peaceful   b) noisy

5) Abstruse
   a) unsure   b) obvious

6) Hasten
   a) dawdle   b) industrious

7) Arrant
   a) array   b) partial

8) Capricious
   a) fickle   b) steadfast

9) Callow
   a) sophisticated   b) jejune

10) Craven
    a) brave   b) coward

11) Cynical
    a) selfish   b) trusting

Answers				
1) Improvement	2) Consistent	3) Genuine	4) Peaceful	5) Obvious
6) Dawdle	7) Partial	8) Steadfast	9) Sophisticated	10) Brave
11) Trusting				

SYNONYMS

The word, 'synonym' has been derived from the Greek word, *syn (with)* and *onoma (name)*. Synonyms are words or expressions with the same or nearly the same meanings. The words may be used as figurative or symbolic substitutes as they have identical meanings. They can be any parts of speech, such as nouns, verbs, adjectives, adverbs or prepositions. A word can have more than one synonym.

Synonyms are very useful. There are times when one avoids repeating the same words over and over again, and it becomes hard to think of an alternative word. A person well equipped with synonyms might not face these problems as the words come handy.

For example:

Synonyms for 'hardworking' are 'diligent', 'determined', 'industrious' and 'enterprising'. Similarly, synonyms for 'beautiful' are pretty, attractive, stunning and lovely and the synonyms for 'kind' are considerate, thoughtful, gracious, amiable, etc.

EXERCISE

The following exercise has three options out of which the reader has to opt for the most apt synonym for each of the given word.

1) Turbulent
   a) violent   b) disturbing   c) difficult

2) Hilarious
   a) amazing   b) depressing   c) humorous

3) Hypocrisy
   a) essential   b) bureaucracy   c) falseness

4) Significant
   a) infirm   b) vital   c) secure

5) Legitimate
   a) critical   b) reliable   c) authorised

6) Obsolete
   a) extinct   b) disordered   c) fragile

7) Embellish
   a) decorate   b) instruct   c) confront

8) Perpetrator
   a) victim   b) culprit   c) prisoner

9) Abandon
   a) leave   b) hate   c) blame

10) Adept
   a) follower   b) believer   c) skilled

11) Consent
   a) accomplish   b) agree   c) fear

12) Vivacious
   a) lively   b) sorrow   c) furious

13) Degrade
   a) loathe   b) ridiculous   c) humiliate

14) Appalling
   a) misgiving   b) neutrality   c) terrifying

15) Despotic
    a) ease   b) arbitrary   c) suitable
16) Apprehend
    a) seize   b) worry   c) adore
17) Elongated
    a) flimsy   b) malleable   c) outstretched
18) Gallop
    a) spring   b) lengthy   c) sprint
19) Obscure
    a) frank   b) peaceful   c) hidden
20) Deceased
    a) unwell   b) misplace   c) dead

Answers				
1) Violent	2) Humorous	3) Falseness	4) Vital	5) Authorized
6) Extinct	7) Decorate	8) Culprit	9) Leave	10) Skilled
11) Agree	12) Lively	13) Humiliate	14) Terrifying	15) Arbitrary
16) Seize	17) Outstretched	18) Sprint	19) Hidden	20) Dead

Choose and tick the correct synonyms of the following words from the options given below the words.

1) Abandon
    a) discard   b) grant   c) plentiful
2) Amenable
    a) misfortunate   b) favorable   c) difficulty
3) Alleviate
    a) rich   b) mitigate   c) vacate
4) Credulous
    a) desire   b) donation   c) confident
5) Baffle
    a) ignore   b) confuse   c) enlarge
6) Fervour
    a) passion   b) squalor   c) nimble
7) Implicate
    a) mammoth   b) candid   c) insinuate

8) Paramount
   a) leading   b) appease   c) exclude

9) Tumult
   a) convey   b) commotion   c) aggressive

10) Sanction
   a) extent   b) distinctive   c) permit

11) Arraign
   a) indict   b) pacify   c) inquire

Answers				
1) Discard	2) Favorable	3) Mitigate	4) Confident	5) Confuse
6) Passion	7) Insinuate	8) Leading	9) Commotion	10) Permit
11) Indict				

CHAPTER 4

HOMOPHONES AND HOMONYMS

The words, 'homophones and homonyms' have originated from the Greek language. Both homophones and homonyms are vastly used in linguistics. *Homophones can be referred to as words that are pronounced the same as another word but have different meanings.* The words may or may not be spelt the same. The words which have different meanings but same pronunciations, and are spelt in the same way are known as *Homonyms*.

For example: Words, such as 'rose' (flower) and 'rose' (past tense of 'rise') are examples of homonyms and words like 'two' and 'to' are examples of homophones.

This topic can be divided into two sections, one consisting of exercise based on homophones and the other on homonyms. The first exercise is based on homophones, where the reader or the student is given two words to fill in the blanks in each sentence and the reader has to choose the correct answer for the correct blank.

EXERCISE

(HOMOPHONES)

1) The eagle's _____ was on a lofty mountain peak in a bright and _____ location.

(airy, aerie)

2) _____ and comfort are accorded to every patient by the nurses _____.

(aide, aid)

3) After we walk down the _____, I'll take you to an _____ of paradise for our honeymoon.

(isle, aisle)

4) The builder was sued for _____ of contract. The labourer dropped his shovel into the _____ of the excavation.

(breach, breech)

5) The _____ of the tree was bent by the wind as if to _____ in homage to nature.

(bow, bough)

6) The wooden _____ had several holes that had been _____ at different times.

(board, bored)

7) The robbers had a hidden _____ of diamonds, jewellery and _____.

(cash, cashe)

8) The supervisor wrote a schedule on the _____ to indicate the days that the operator should oil the _____.

(calender, calendar)

9) What _____ to the beauty of subtractive wood sculpting, is the careful use of the _____.

(adds, adz)

10) One should _____ a will or reveal the contents of _____ a death that may   exclude an unnamed _____.

(ere, heir, air)

11) After the _____ had laboured to complete the poetry, the   authorities _____ it from the recital.

(bard, barred)

12) The church _____ attracted many strangers, some of   them dressed and acted in _____ ways.

(bizarre, bazaar)

13) Her loving _____ brought a _____ for her hair.

(beau, bow)

14) The _____ winds through the valley made all the doors _____ of the house _____.

(creek, creak)

Answers

1) Aerie, airy	2) Aid, aide	3) Aisle, isle	4) Breach, breech
5) Bough, bow	6) Board, bored	7) Cahse, cash	8) Calendar, calendar
9) Adds, adz	10) Air, ere, heir	11) Bard, barred	12) Bazaar, bizarre
13) Beau, bow	14) Creek, creak	15) Principal, principle	

Fill in the blanks with the correct homophones from the options given within the brackets.

1) The _____ played such cacophonous music throughout the performance that it was _____ from further auditions.

(banned, band)

2) The lower _____ of a railroad sleeper car was the only available place for her to give _____ to the baby.

(berth, birth)

3) With confused expressions, the book sales persons furrowed their _____ when the student proceeded to _____ through every book in the store.

(brows, browse)

4) Have you read the story about the tortoise and the _____?

(hair, hare)

5) The _____ flew overhead and screeched _____!

(awk, auk)

6) When the _____ bounced over the fence and out of reach, the child began to _____ and sob.

(bawl, ball)

7) He had to _____ the drums for four hours before he was entitled to a dinner which included an entree, a _____ salad and a beverage.

(beat, beet)

Answers

1) Band, banned		2) Berth, birth	3) Brows, browse	4) Hare
5) Auk, awk	6) Ball, bawl	7) Beat, beet		

(HOMONYMS)

This one is a guessing exercise based on homonyms. The given sentences are clues to the oneword answers which have the same pronunciations and spellings but different meanings. The word in each case should be appropriate to make sense for both the sentences as they are in different contexts.

1) Opposite for hit/Mr., Mrs., _____.

2) A musical instrument you blow/two of these can be found on a bull's head.

3) A place with lots of games and rides/to treat people without favouritism.

4) Opposite of right/past tense of leave.

5) Child / baby goat/to trick someone.

6) You can wear these to help you see better/you can serve drinks in them.

7) The substance used to make tyres/something used to erase pencil.

8) A container/type of plant/to fight with fists.

9) Not moving/continuing to do something.

10) To look after something/your brain.

11) You hit one with a hammer/there is one on the end of every finger.

12) To fire a gun/a new growth on a plant.

13) A boy's name/a teacher can _____ your work.

14) Opposite of hot/if you catch one you sneeze.

15) A month/could

16) You have to pay this for doing wrong/the weather can be _____(sunny)

17) A place where someone is buried/serious _____

18) You can _____ your name/you can make a_____ with your hand

19) You can kick, throw, or catch this/Cindrella went to one.

20) You strike this to get a flame/you can have a football _____.

Answers				
1) Miss	2) Horn	3) Fair	4) Left	5) Kid
6) Glasses	7) Rubber	8) Box	9) Still	10) Mind
11) Nail	12) Shoot	13) Mark	14) Cold	15) May
16) Fine	17) Grave	18) Sign	19) Ball	20) Match

CHAPTER 5

PREFIX AND SUFFIX

Prefixes and Suffixes are widely used in order to form new words or to alter the meanings of the words by adding a group of letters before or after each word. The group of letters added in front of the word is known as *prefix* and the group of letters added at the end of the word is known as *suffix*.

The exercise below will target on readers' skills of analysing each word. The reader has been provided with a word and its meaning, and one has to add a prefix or a suffix to the word in order to alter the meaning.

For example:

He was acting in a very _____ way. (child)

Answer-childish

Where 'child' is the **noun** or the **main word** and 'ish' is the **suffix**, as it comes after the main word. Similarly,

Example:

Gandiji fought against _____. (touchability)

Where 'touchability' is the **main word** and 'un' is the **prefix**, as it comes before the main word.

1) He was sitting _____ in his seat on the train. (comfort)

EXERCISE

2) Some of the shanty towns are dreadfully _____. (crowd)

3) This word is very difficult to spell, and even worse, it's _____. (pronounce)

4) You need to be a highly trained _____ to understand this report. (economy)

5) There were only a _____ of people at the match. (hand)

6) He wants to be a _____ when he grows up. (mathematics)

7) They had to _____ the lion before they could catch it. (tranquil)

8) You need a _____ of motivation, organisation and revision to learn English. (combine)

9) His _____ has been expected for the last half an hour. (arrive)

10) She had no _____ of going to see him. (intend)

11) Failing her driving test was a great _____ to her. (appoint)

12) He decided to study _____ at university. (journal)

13) With the real plan, the rate of _____ in Brazil has fallen. (inflate)

14) The party was _____ , everything went wrong. (disaster)

15) The event was totally _____ . It was terrible. (organised)

16) He was _____ . He wouldn't change his mind. (compromise)

17) He spent half an hour _____ himself with the building. (familiar)

18) She looked at her _____ in the mirror. (reflect)

19) The team that he supported were able to win the_____ . (champion)

20) He didn't pass his exam. He was _____ for the second time. (succeed)

Answers

1) Comfortably	2) Crowded	3) Pronunciation	4) Economist	5) Handful
6) Mathematician	7) Tranquilize	8) Combination	9) Arrival	10) Intentions
11) Disappointment	12) Journalism	13) Inflation	14) Disastrous	15) Unorganized
16) Compromising	17) Familiarising	18) Reflection	19) Championship	20) Unsuccessful

IDIOMS, PROVERBS & PHRASES

A combination of words which have figurative meanings are called *idioms or phrases*. These are expressions which are often metaphorical and separate from the literal meaning or definition of words. There are numerous idioms and phrases used in our everyday conversations making the language more colourful.

For example:

a) *Piece of cake*:
    something which is very easy.

b) *Dress to kill*:
    to wear one's finest clothes.

c) *Adding fuel to the fire*:
    to make a bad situation even worse.

EXERCISE

(IDIOMS)

The first exercise below is based on idioms. There will be various idioms from which the reader has to choose the correct idiom to fill in each of the blanks in the following sentences.

i.   Barking up the wrong tree
ii.   Out of the blue
iii. Fly by the seat of her pants
iv.   Like a third wheel
v.   Get his act together
vi.   Off his rocker
vii. Butterflies in my stomach
viii. Like the pot calling the kettle black
ix.   Get a word in edgewise
x.   Off in the clouds
xi.   Some song and dance
xii. Hit the roof
xiii. Throw the book at him
xiv. Chickens with their heads cut off
xv.   Blow off some steam
xvi. Burn the midnight oil
xvii. In the red
xviii. Searching for a needle in the haystack
xix. Burning the candle at both ends
xx.   Run circles around

Answers				
1) v	2) xii	3) iv	4) xi	5) xiii
6) xx	7) vii	8) xiv	9) vi	10) i
11) xv	12) xix	13) xvi	14) xviii	15) viii
16) ii	17) xvii	18) x	19) iii	20) ix

Choose the correct idiom or phrase for each of the following sentences:

1) If he doesn't_____, he'll be forced to leave the school.
2) My boss will _____if those papers are not found.
3) At dinner with my roommate and his girlfriend, I felt_____.
4) He gave us _____about why the work wasn't finished.
5) This is his third offense and the police should _____.
6) Our offense was able to _____around their defense.
7) Before giving my speech in front of the whole class, I had _____.
8) When the lunchroom is busy, the cafeteria workers run around _____.
9) After giving that crazy lecture that made no sense, we thought our teacher was_____.
10) If you think that I stole your jacket, you're_____.
11) Physical exercise is a good way to_____.
12) Instead of_____, you need to cut back on some of your activities and commitments.
13) During the week of final exams, many students will _____.
14) Finding a contact lens on a crowded dance floor is like _____.
15) Dad accusing you of eating too much is like the _____.
16) One day, _____, I got a call from a friend I hadn't heard from in years.
17) How does he pay the bills when his business is always_____?
18) He seldom pays attention in class and it seems that his head is _____.
19) Finding the student unprepared for class, the teacher had to _____.
20) He didn't use complete sentences until he was 4 years old, but then no one could _____.

Answers				
1) q	2) m	3) a	4) h	5) n
6) i	7) e	8) d	9) g	10) b
11) l	12) j	13) t	14) s	15) r
16) o	17) p	18) k	19) f	

(PHRASES)

A group of words within a sentence or a clause is referred to as *phrases*. The phrase functions as a unit and includes a head which determines the type or nature of the phrase.

For example:

When this is all over, your father might be ***going away*** for a little while.

Here ***going away*** is the phrase telling the nature of the sentence i.e., phrasal verb.

Fill in the blanks using the appropriate phrase from the options given below the sentences in each case:

1) You must _____ and make plans for the future.

    a) Look on   b) Look up

    c) Look ahead   d) Look back

2) There were so many panes of glass broken that the windows couldn't _____ the rain.

    a) keep on   b) keep up

    c) keep out   d) keep back

3) Children have a natural inclination to look _____ to their parents.

    a) Forward to   b) Up to

    c) Out on   d) Back to

4) He looks _____ me because I spend my holidays in *India* instead of going abroad.

    a) Down at   b) Down on

    c) Out of   d) Back on

5) The crowd _____ while the police surrounded the house.

    a) Looked on   b) Looked up

    c) Looked out   d) Looked at

6) I had to wait for permission from the Town Council before I could _____ with my plans.

    a) Go round   b) Go up

    c) Go on   d) Go back

7) He _____ his mother; he has blue eyes and fair hair.

    a) Takes out   b) Takes up

    c) Takes on   d) Takes after

8) Don't _____ with the idea that Scotsmen are mean. They just don't like wasting money.

    a) Run out   b) Run away

    c) Run on   d) Run off

9) I _____ to an old school friend in the tube today.
   a) Ran in
   b) Ran up
   c) Ran on
   d) Ran off

10) I _____ Tom in chess and beat him.
    a) Took out
    b) Took up
    c) Took on
    d) Took off

11) As a parent, you should _____ such small mistakes from the kids.
    a) Allow into
    b) Allow for
    c) Allow with
    d) Make allowances

12) The principal became furious on hearing the news of the students' unrest but eventually _____.
    a) calmed into
    b) calmed down
    c) calmed over
    d) calmed up

13) For the sake of his health, Siddhu decided to _____ smoking.
    a) Give through
    b) Give along
    c) Give up
    d) Give for

14) The teacher requested the class representative to _____ the answer sheets to all the students.
    a) Hand at
    b) Hand on
    c) Hand back
    d) Hand out

15) Tina eagerly _____ the day her exams would get over and she would be back to partying with her friends.
    a) Looked forward to
    b) Looked after
    c) Looked up to
    d) Looked down on

16) It took the firemen a long time to _____ the blazing fire.
    a) Put off
    b) Put out
    c) Put on
    d) Put up

17) I wanted to _____ the dress before buying it, in order to check if it was the right size for me.
    a) Rely on
    b) Take on
    c) Look on
    d) Try on

18) Aisha _____ her mother to a great degree.
    a) Takes off
    b) Took out
    c) Takes on
    d) Takes after

19) The policeman was quick to _____ the number of the speeding car.
    a) Back down
    b) Calm down

c) Note down   d) Let down

20) After the movie got over, she decided to _____ with her friends till the evening.

a) Hang out   b) Hang up

c) Hurry up   d) Iron out

Answers				
1) c	2) c	3) b	4) b	5) a
6) c	7) d	8) b	9) a	10) c
11) b	12) b	13) c	14) d	15) a
16) b	17) d	18) d	19) c	20) a

(PROVERBS)

Proverbs, on the other hand are short and pithy sayings which express wisdom or advice and some traditionally held truth. These statements are metaphorical in nature and are transmitted from generation to generation.

For example:

a)   Where there's a will there's a way:

when a person really wants to do something, he will find a way of doing it no matter what.

b)   All that glitters is not gold:

Do not be deceived by things or offers that appear to be attractive.

The reader has to find the right proverb from the given choices in each case and match them with their meanings given below:

1)   Uneasy lies the head that wears the crown.
2)   Wake not a sleeping lion.
3)   Waste not, want not.
4)   Where ignorance is bliss, it is folly to be wise.
5)   The wish is the father to the thought.
6)   Nothing ventured, nothing gained.
7)   Every ass likes to hear himself bray.
8)   The apple doesn't fall far from the tree.
9)   Still waters run deep.
10)   The die is cast.
11)   The road to hell is paved with good intentions.
12)   Time and tide wait for no man.
13)   Two wrongs don't make a right.
14)   Virtue is its own reward.
15)   The end justifies the means.

Meanings:

i.   Children resemble their parents.
ii.   If one is careful with things especially money, one will not lack them when needed.
iii.   It is wrong to harm someone because they have harmed you.
iv.   You should not expect praise for acting in a correct or moral way.
v.   Without risks, there are no rewards.
vi.   Wrong or unfair methods may be used if the result of the action is good.
vii.   A quiet person can have much knowledge or wisdom.
viii. One must not miss opportunities by delaying action.

ix. With greatness and power comes a lot of responsibilities.
x. It is not enough to intend to do something , you must actually do it.
xi. Foolish people talk a lot.
xii. It is wise not to disturb things at times lest you invite trouble.
xiii. The decision has been made and its impossible to change.
xiv. You think that something is true because you want it to be so.
xv. It is better to be unaware of something that will bring unhappiness.

Answers

1) ix	2) xii	3) ii	4) xv	5) xiv
6) v	7) xi	8) i	9) vii	10) xiii
11) x	12) viii	13) iii	14) iv	15) vi

Chapter 2

ONE-WORD SUBSTITUTES

One word can often express the idea of a phrase or clause and can help in writing or communicating precisely. Some common one-word substitutes are given below. Please learn them thoroughly to improve your word power or vocabulary.

1. A name and opted by a writer = Pseudonym
2. Of unknown authorship = Anonymous
3. Taking one's own life = Suicide
4. A person concerned with practical results = Pragmatist
5. A speech by an actor at the end of a play = Epilogue
6. A political leader who tries to stir up people = Demagogue
7. Animals living on land and in water = Amphibians
8. A person with long experience = Veteran
9. Atonement for one's sins = Repentance
10. A man of odd habits = Eccentric
11. A person who derives pleasure by inflicting pain on others = Sadist
12. A general pardon of political offender = Amnesty
13. A person who is made to bear the blame due to others = Scapegoat
14. A person who pays much attention to his clothes and appearance = Dandy
15. A person hard to please = Fastidious
16. A person who considers himself superior to others in culture and intellect = Highbrow
17. A wishful longing for something one has known in the past = Nostalgia
18. The art of cutting trees and bushes in to ornamental shapes = Topiary
19. An associate in an office or institution = Colleague
20. A person who believes in God = Theist
21. A person who does not believe in God = Atheist
22. Witty, Clever, Retort = Repartee
23. A child who stays away from school without any good reason = Truant
24. One who compiles a dictionary = Lexicographer
25. One who does not care for literature and art = Philistine

26. One who totally abstains from alcoholic drinks = Teetotaller

27. A house for storing grains = Granary

28. A person who is neither intelligent nor dull (average) = Mediocre

29. A person who dances to the tune of his wife = Henpecked

30. A branch of medicine which deals with the problems of the old = Geriatrics

31. Careful in performing duties = Punctilious

32. A person who gives written testimony for use in a law court = Deponent

33. Equal in rank, merit or quality = Peer

34. Indifference to pleasure or pain = Stoicism

35. Using of new words = Coinage

36. Fruit garden = Orchard

37. Person who gives himself up to luxury and sexual pleasures = Voluptuary

38. Books which excite sex in readers = Pornography

39. One who is likable = Amiable

40. One who copies the writing of others = Plagiarist (Plagiarism)

41. A journey to a holy place = Pilgrimage

42. Worship of idols = Idolatry

43. One who ruins the statues of gods = Iconoclast

44. One who is honourably discharged from service = Emeritus

45. A place of ideal peace and happiness = Elysium

46. Printed notice of somebody's death = Obituary

47. A story in verse = Ballad

48. One knowing everything = Omniscient

49. One who is present everywhere = Omnipresent

50. One who is all powerful = Omnipotent

ACRONYMS

An acronym or abbreviation is formed by taking the initial letters or group of letters taken from a word or series of words, that is itself pronounced as a word.

Such as ROM – Read Only Memory

ATM – At This Moment

AWA – As Well As

PTO – Please Turn Over

DYK – Do You Know

UNO – United Naitons Organisation

WHO – World Health Organisation

EXERCISE

Below are a few commonly used acronyms and the reader has to write the full form against each of them.

1) RADAR
2) NAAFI
3) NASA
4) LASER
5) SCUBA
6) UNESCO
7) AIDS
8) SAT

9) PIN
10) RAM
11) RSVP
12) ESL/EFL
13) AM/PM
14) AD/BC
15) ASAP

Answers

1) Radio Detection and Ranging
2) Navy, Army and Air Force Institutes
3) National Aeronautics and Space Administration
4) Light Amplification through Stimulated Emission of Radiation
5) Self-Contained Underwater Breathing Apparatus
6) United Nations Educational, Scientific and Cultural Organization
7) Acquired Immune Deficiency Syndrome
8) Scholastic Assessment Test
9) Personal Identification Number
10) Random Access Memory
11) Responder sil uous plait – (French) meaning 'Please respond'
12) English as Second Language/English Foreign Language
13) Ante Meridian (before noon)/Post Meridian (after noon)
14) Anno Domini (Lalen) – (In the year of our Laord)/Before Christ
15) As Sooon As Possible

Given below are a few commonly used acronyms and the reader has to write the full form against each of them.

1) Maser
2) Internet
3) Sonar
4) SWAT
5) BASIC
6) BIOS
7) AHEAD
8) STEPS
9) UNICEF
10) UNESCO

Answers

1) Molecular Amplification by Stimulated Emission of Radiations
2) International Network
3) Sound navigation and ranging
4) Special Weapons and Tactics
5) Beginners All-purpose Symbolic Instruction Code
6) Basic Input/Output System
7) Association on Higher Education and Disability
8) Sequenced Transition to Education in the Public Schools
9) United Nations International Children's Emergency Fund.
10) United Nations Educational, Scientific and Cultural Organization

SELF IMPROVEMENT/PERSONALITY DEVELOPMENT

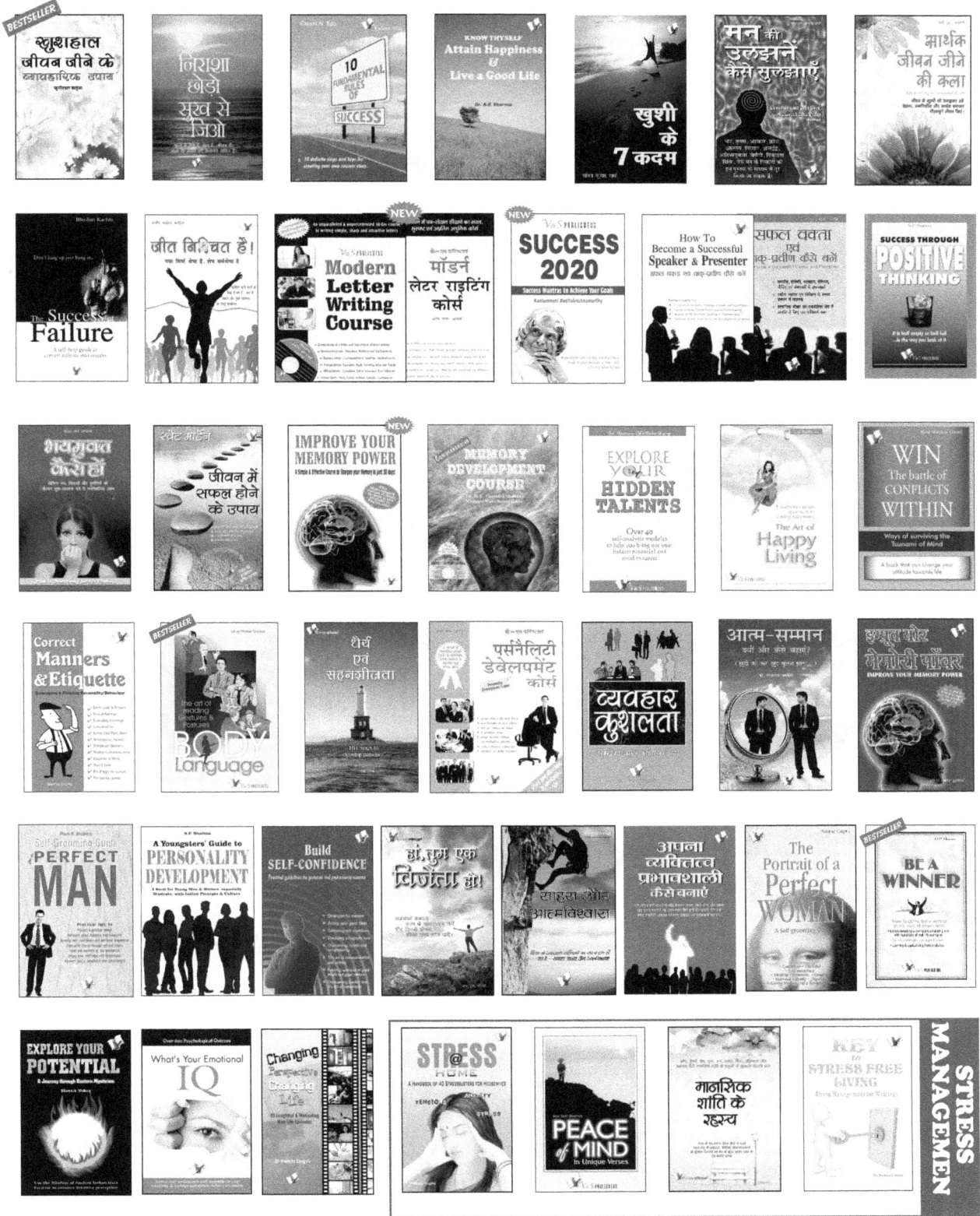

All books available at www.vspublishers.com

QUIZ BOOKS

ENGLISH IMPROVEMENT

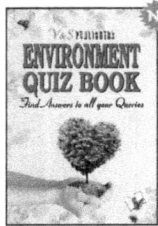

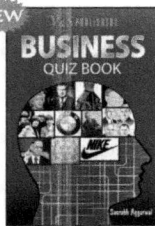

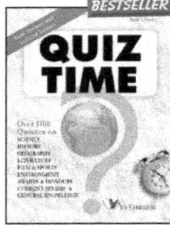

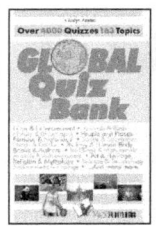

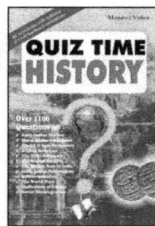

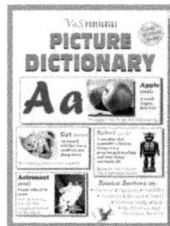

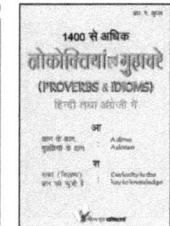

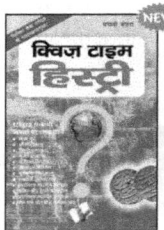

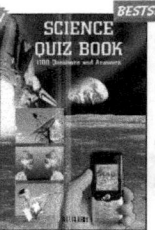

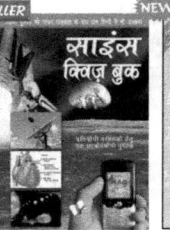

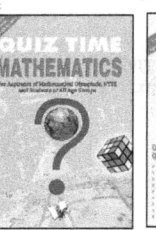

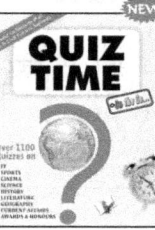

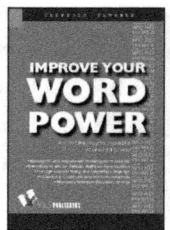

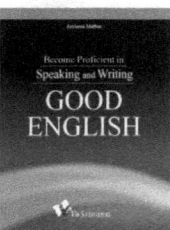

OTHERS LANGUAGE

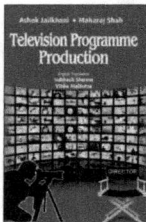

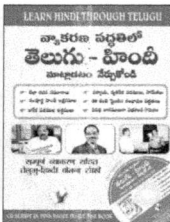

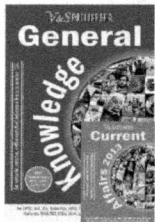

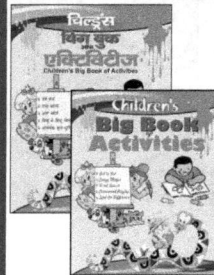

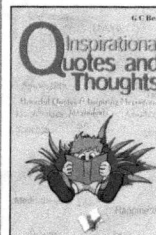

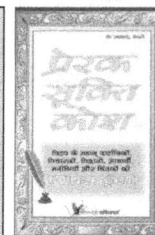

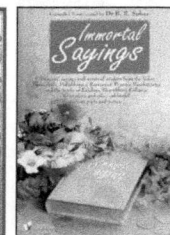

ACTIVITIES BOOK

QUOTES/SAYINGS

BIOGRAPHIES/CHILDREN SCIENCE LIBRARY

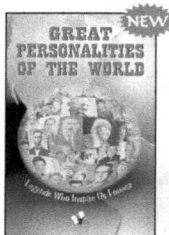

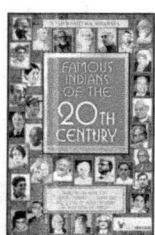

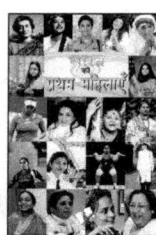

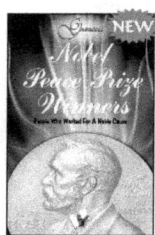

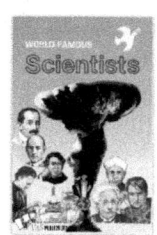

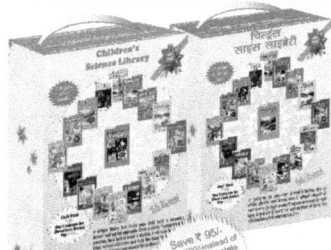

Set Code: 02122 S

COMPUTER BOOKS

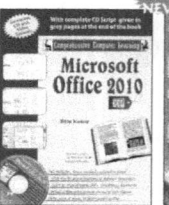

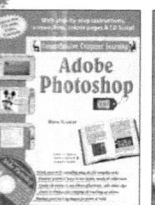

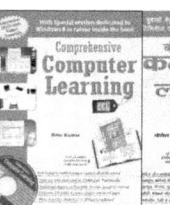

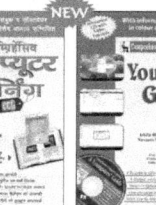

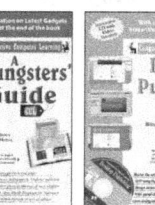

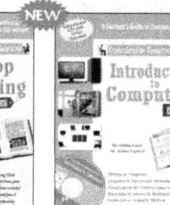

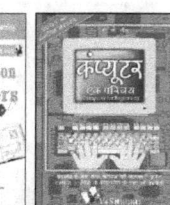

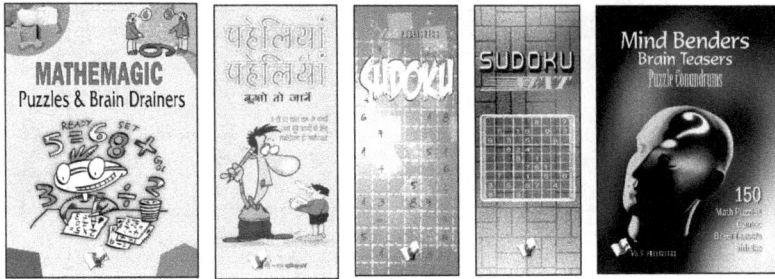

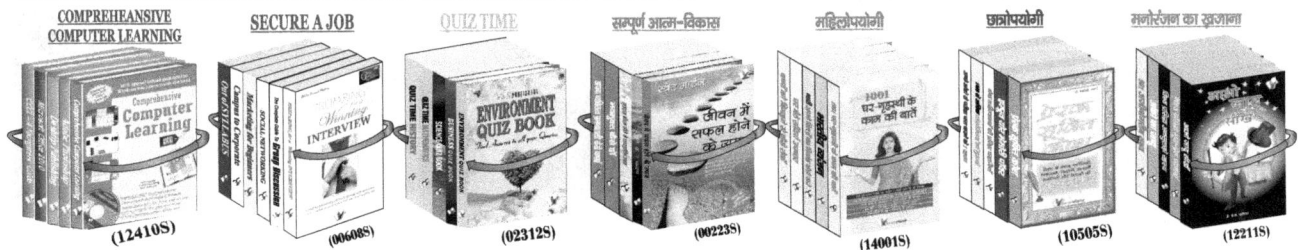

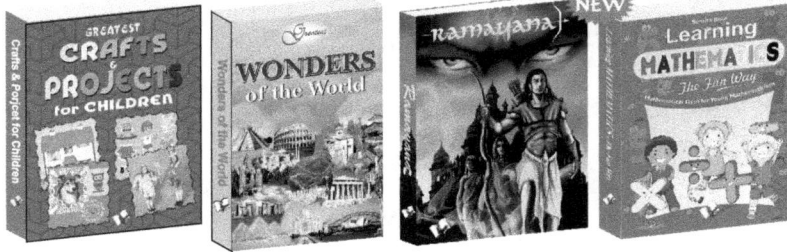

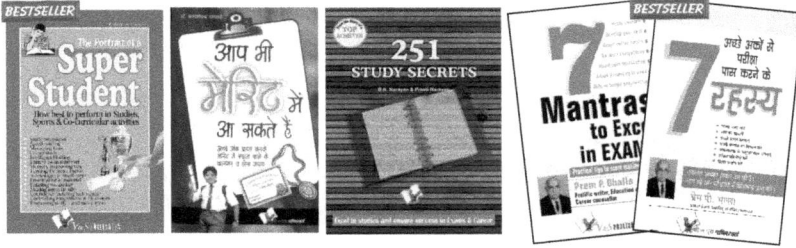

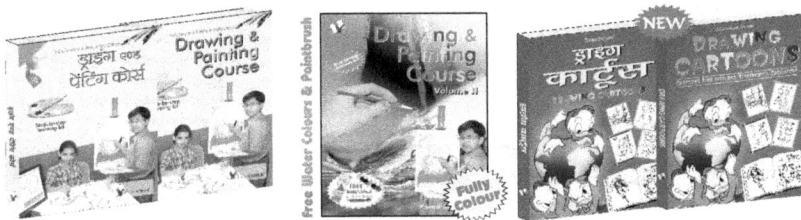

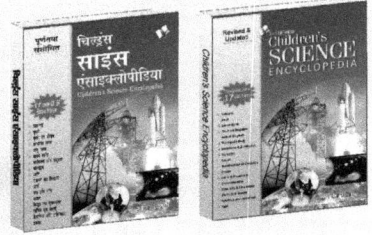

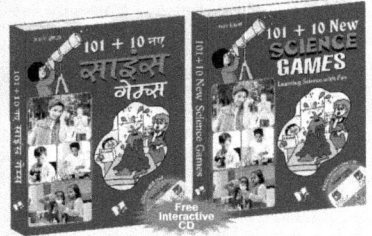

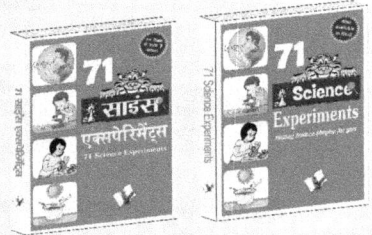

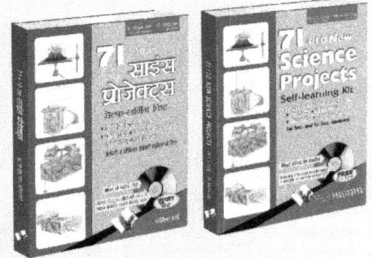

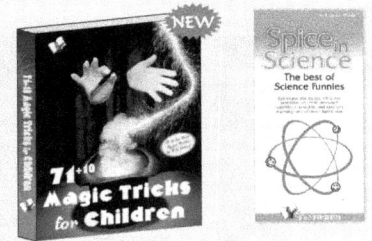

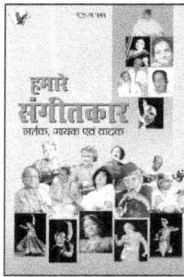

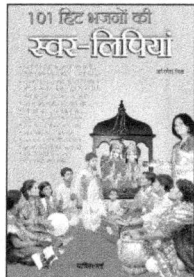

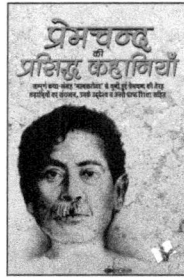

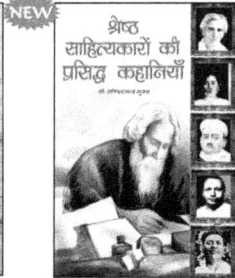

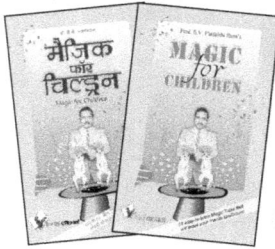

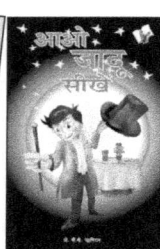

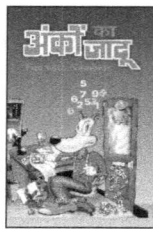

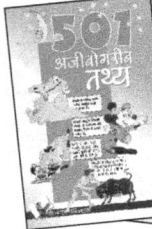

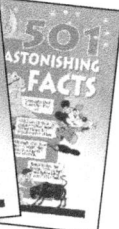

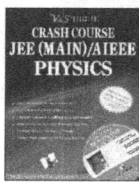

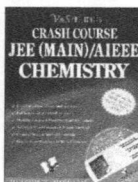

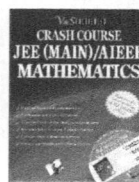

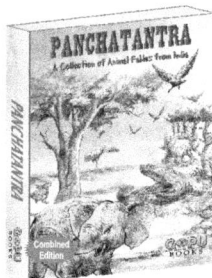

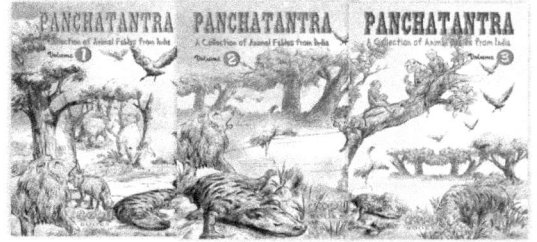

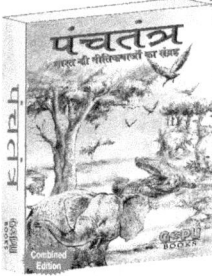

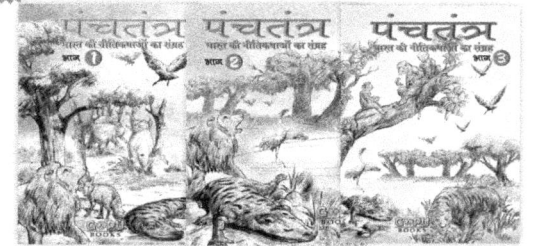

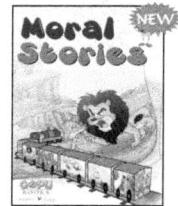

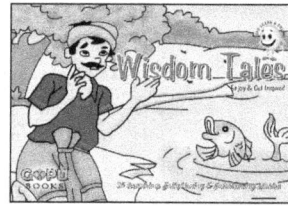

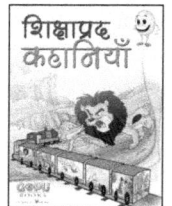

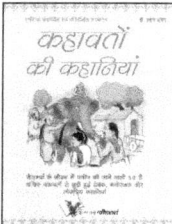

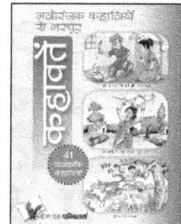

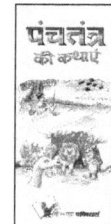

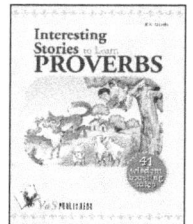

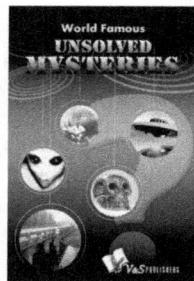

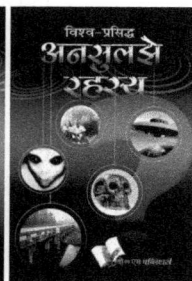

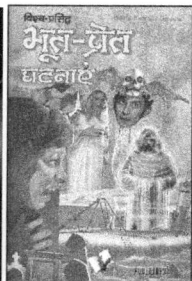

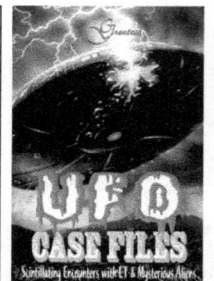

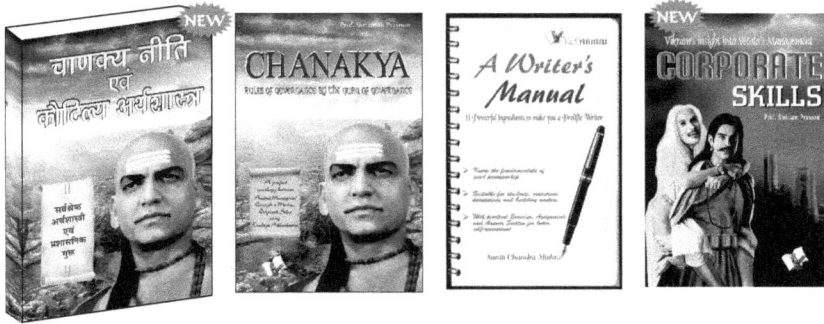

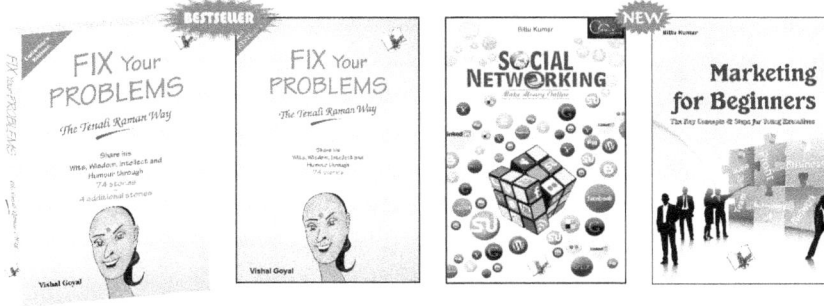

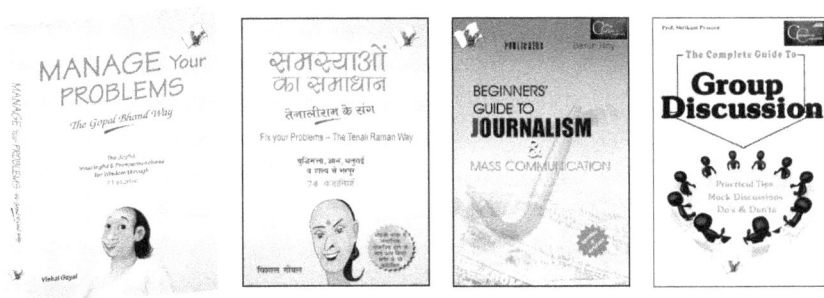

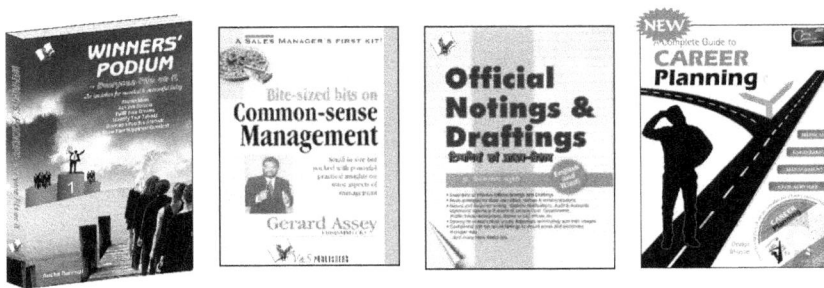

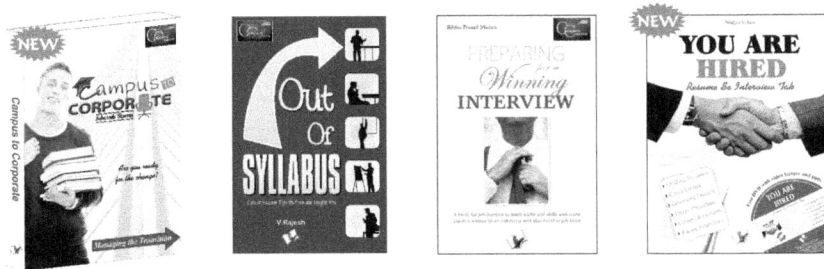

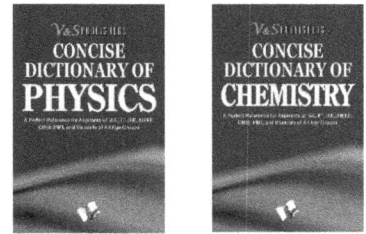

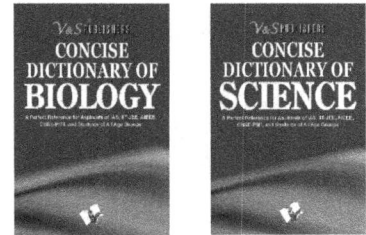

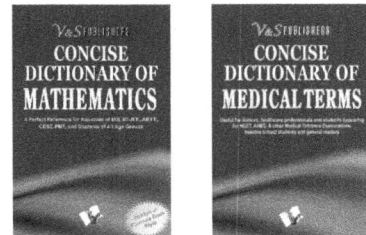

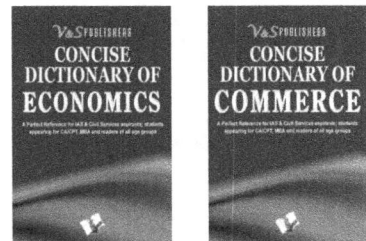

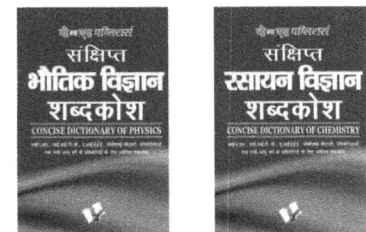

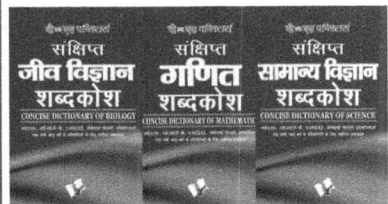

www.ingramcontent.com/pod-product-compliance
Lightning Source LLC
Chambersburg PA
CBHW080233270326
41926CB00020B/4225